Canada's Everyday
Diabetes Choice
Recipes

Edited by
Katherine E. Younker
MBA, RD, Certified Diabetes Educator

Published in cooperation with

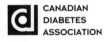

CANADIAN DIABETES ASSOCIATION | ASSOCIATION CANADIENNE DU DIABÈTE

Robert ROSE

For a list of contributing authors, see page 183.
For complete cataloguing information, see page 184.

Disclaimer
The recipes in this book have been carefully tested by our kitchen and our tasters. To the best
of our knowledge, they are safe and nutritious for ordinary use and users. For those people
with food or other allergies, or who have special food requirements or health issues, please read
the suggested contents of each recipe carefully and determine whether or not they may create
a problem for you. All recipes are used at the risk of the consumer.

We cannot be responsible for any hazards, loss or damage that may occur as a result of any
recipe use.

For those with special needs, allergies, requirements or health problems, in the event of
any doubt, please contact your medical adviser prior to the use of any recipe.

Design & Production: PageWave Graphics Inc.
Photography: Mark T. Shapiro

The publisher and editor wish to express their appreciation to the following supplier of props
used in the cover photography:

DISHES AND LINENS
Homefront
371 Eglinton Ave. W.
Toronto, Ontario M5N 1A3
Tel: (416) 488-3189
www.homefrontshop.com

Cover image: Chicken, Red Pepper and Snow Pea Stir-Fry (see recipe, page 72)

We acknowledge the financial support of the Government of Canada through the
Book Publishing Industry Development Program (BPIDP) for our publishing activities.

Published by: Robert Rose Inc.
120 Eglinton Ave. E., Suite 1000, Toronto, Ontario, Canada M4P 1E2
Tel: (416) 322-6552   Fax: (416) 322-6936

Printed in Canada

1 2 3 4 5 6 7 8 9 10   GP   09 08 07 06 05 04 03

Contents

Foreword

Canada's Everyday Diabetes Choice Recipes is a collection of recipes from a variety of authors. It reflects the wealth of cooking styles and foods used across Canada.

Anyone involved in diabetes care knows that dietary intake is a key factor in delaying the onset of, and managing, diabetes. Studies have shown this time and again. This collection of recipes provides you and your family with many great dishes, along with information on how to include them in a healthy lifestyle.

More and more Canadians are being diagnosed with diabetes or some form of glucose intolerance every day. Good nutrition and healthy eating together with an active lifestyle are keys to successfully managing blood glucose levels, while reducing the risk for other chronic diseases such as cardiovascular disease, osteoporosis and cancer.

All recipes in this book have been analyzed for nutrient content and on each page you will find the nutrient information (energy in calories, carbohydrate, fiber, protein, fat, saturated fat, cholesterol, and sodium) to help you include these recipes in a healthy lifestyle or fit them into your meal plan.

The **Canadian Diabetes Association Food Choice Values and Symbols** system is provided for those who follow a meal plan and use the Good Health Eating Guide. **Carbohydrate and fiber** have been included with each recipe to permit easy carbohydrate counting for those who like more flexibility at meals. Whatever method you choose to provide yourself with great nutrition, these recipes are for you.

Recipe tips, make-ahead information and suggestions for completing meals are also included. You are sure to find new spins on some of your family's favorites and other recipes that will soon become standards. I hope you will find this a welcome addition to your healthy lifestyle.

— Kathy

On Managing Diabetes

The Canadian Diabetes Association reports that one in 13 people have diabetes and statistics worldwide report that diabetes is growing at epidemic proportions. Recent health studies have focused on identifying risk factors and looking at how to slow the epidemic. Health Canada now recommends that a combination of good nutrition and physical activity can actually help reduce the risk or postpone the development of type 2 diabetes." (See www.healthcanada.ca/diabetes.)

There are many risk factors for diabetes. If you or a family member has diabetes, examining these risk factors may help prevent or postpone type 2 diabetes in other family members. The degree of your risk can be determined by your answers to these questions:

- **Do I have a family member with diabetes?**
  There is an increased risk of type 2 diabetes in families with a history of diabetes.

  One preventative strategy is to ensure that other family members are screened to detect any elevated glucose levels early.

- **How old am I?**
  The risk of getting type 2 diabetes increases with age. All people over age 40 should be screened according to recommended guidelines. The risk of developing diabetes increases with every decade lived until the 80s. The longer you live, the greater your chances of developing diabetes.

- **Am I a woman who has given birth to a child weighing over 9 lbs (4 kg)?**
  Having a large birth weight baby may be a risk factor for developing type 2 diabetes later in life. Gestational diabetes, which occurs in 2-4% of all pregnancies, increases the risk for developing type 2 diabetes 5 to 20 years after this pregnancy. Women who have had a baby weighing over 9 lbs at birth may have had undetected gestational diabetes. Additional pregnancies further increase the risk of developing type 2 diabetes, as each added pregnancy places more strain on the pancreas. Children born to mothers who have had gestational diabetes during that pregnancy are also at increased risk of developing type 2 diabetes later in life.

- **Am I overweight?**
  Overweight and obesity are common health problems worldwide. Studies have shown that 80% of people with type 2 diabetes are overweight. The risk is greater when the extra weight is located around the middle. Reducing body weight by as little as 5–7% can prevent or delay the development of diabetes when added to regular physical activity.

Other risk factors include:
- history of impaired fasting glucose or impaired glucose tolerance
- member of a high-risk population (Aboriginal, Asian, African or Hispanic)
- the presence of high blood pressure
- the presence of elevated blood fat levels (high cholesterol or triglycerides)
- the presence of any disease of the blood vessels (vascular disease)
- in women, the presence of polycystic ovarian disease
- the presence of any complication related to diabetes (like heart disease).

Preventing and Managing Diabetes

Preventing Diabetes

Eating a balanced low-fat diet, including high-fiber carbohydrate choices and moderate portion sizes can help to promote a healthy weight, and when coupled together with regular physical activity can help reduce the risk of diabetes for the population at large.

Recent studies have also shown that appropriate dietary intake can improve blood glucose levels significantly. Activity can further decrease blood glucose levels and increase the body's sensitivity to insulin.

How much activity is enough?
Health Canada reports that "A brisk walk for 30 minutes, or similar activity, five times a week, can lower the risk of developing type 2 diabetes." (www.healthcanada.ca/diabetes) Active living is integral to the lives of people of ALL ages. Those adults over the age of 60, with the highest prevalence of type 2 diabetes, have been found to benefit positively from increasing their daily physical activity.

Managing diabetes

Once diagnosed, managing diabetes requires daily attention. Food intake, activity, blood glucose monitoring and healthy lifestyle choices are all part of the package.

Current recommendations for blood glucose targets are lower than ever and closer to the recommendations for those without diabetes. Studies have shown that risk for developing all types of diabetes complications increases proportionately to the elevation in blood glucose levels. For those with diabetes, blood glucose targets are 4–7 mmol/L before meals and 5–10 mmol/L 2 hours after eating. For those without diabetes, normal ranges are 4–6 mmol/L before meals and 5–8 mmol/L 2 hours after.

Nutrition Principles for Canadians with Diabetes

Canada's Guidelines for Healthy Eating apply to all Canadians including those with diabetes. These guidelines are:

1. Enjoy a VARIETY of foods.
2. Emphasize cereals, breads, other grain products, vegetables and fruit.
3. Choose lower-fat dairy products, leaner meats and food prepared with little or no fat.
4. Achieve and maintain a healthy body weight by enjoying regular physical activity and healthy eating.
5. Limit salt, alcohol and caffeine.

More detailed recommendations for people with diabetes Canada come from the *The Guidelines for the Nutritional Management of Diabetes Mellitus in the New Millennium: A Position Statement by the Canadian Diabetes Association.*

Carbohydrate

Recommendations regarding carbohydrate indicate that 50–60% of energy (calories) should be obtained from carbohydrate sources including starch foods, vegetables, fruits, milk products and added sugar. Added sugars, (sucrose, fructose, glucose, etc.) as opposed to those found in vegetables, fruit and milk products may comprise up to 10% of energy intake.

Fiber

A fiber intake of at least 25-35 g a day is recommended. High-fiber food choices are preferred, particularly those with a low glycemic index (see page 17). Fiber should be chosen from a variety of sources and it is suggested that choosing at least 5–10 g from soluble fiber sources can help to reduce serum (blood) cholesterol.

Protein

Recommendations regarding protein suggest a moderate intake with some emphasis on vegetable protein sources such as beans, lentils and soybeans.

Fat

In keeping with recommendations for all Canadians, an intake of less than 30% of energy from fat, and less than 10% from saturated fat, is recommended. A high fat intake can increase the risk of cardiovascular disease by helping to raise blood lipids (cholesterol), promote weight gain and impair glucose tolerance. Intake of processed foods containing saturated and trans fats should be limited. Monounsaturated fats (from canola, olive and peanut oil) are recommended where possible and polyunsaturated fat should be limited to less than 10% of fat (see page 11).

Alcohol

An alcohol intake of less than 5% of energy or less than two drinks per day (fewer than 14 regular drinks per week for men and fewer than 9 per week for women) is suggested. Use of alcohol should be discussed with the diabetes health care team, as it can further aggravate conditions such as hypertension (high blood pressure), dyslipidemia (high blood fat levels) and liver function. Consumption of alcohol can cause either hyperglycemia (high blood glucose) or hypoglycemia (low blood sugar). Due to the risk of hypoglycemia it is recommended that people with diabetes consume a source of carbohydrate with alcohol. They should also inform family and friends regarding the risk and wear identification such as a medic alert bracelet.

Sweeteners

Both sweeteners in the form of "nutritive" (sugar, fructose, aspartame and sugar alcohols) and "non-nutritive" (acesulfame potassium, sucralose, saccharin and cyclamate) can play roles in the diet of the person with diabetes. Sugar alcohols such as sorbitol, xylitol, mannitol, maltitol, lactitol and isomalt, may be used in moderation with little effect on blood glucose (sugar) levels. In large amounts, they may cause flatulence (gas) and diarrhea. Health Canada has provided an acceptable daily intake for aspartame and the "non-nutritive" sweeteners acesulfame potassium, sucralose, saccharin and cyclamate. These amounts are based on body weight and for most individuals with diabetes, moderate use of these sweeteners is acceptable. Discuss sweetener use with the dietitian on your diabetes health care team. For more information on sweeteners see the Canadian Diabetes Association website: www.diabetes.ca .

Vitamins and Minerals

The recommended intake of vitamins and minerals for people with diabetes is the same as for all Canadians. Most individuals can obtain adequate amounts of these nutrients by consuming a well-balanced diet. When vitamins and minerals are obtained from plant sources, other components in the plant called "phytochemicals" are consumed as well. These "phytochemicals" are also thought to protect against disease.

Reducing Sodium

Many people with diabetes also have hypertension (elevated blood pressure). Reducing sodium intake is one way to lower blood pressure. Salt (or sodium chloride) contains about 2400 mg of sodium per teaspoon. Reducing sodium intake to 2000 to 4000 mg can help to reduce blood pressure levels in those individuals who are salt sensitive. There are several ways to reduce the sodium in your diet:

- Avoid using the salt shaker on the table.
- Modify your recipes: Avoid adding salt and where appropriate substitute herbs, spices or flavored vinegars.
- Read the nutrition labels on packages and choose products which are lower in sodium.
- Use reduced-sodium or no-salt-added products, such as reduced-sodium soya sauce, teriyaki sauce, MSG and other condiments.
- Choose low-sodium soup mixes or make your own.
- Choose whole, fresh, unprocessed foods and avoid canned and convenience ones where possible. If you choose canned products such as vegetables, drain and rinse the liquid from the food before using.
- Avoid processed meats (such as weiners and ham) or choose sodium-reduced types.
- Limit foods packed in brines such as pickles, sauerkraut, olives etc.
- Choose crackers and snack foods which are reduced in sodium.
- Reduce your use of condiments such as mustard, horseradish, ketchup, and Worcestershire sauce.

The Canadian Diabetes Association recommends that all persons with diabetes receive nutrition counselling from a registered dietitian. Work with your diabetes health care team to review your dietary intake and develop a meal plan which will best suit your lifestyle. Ask your physician for a reference or call your local Diabetes Center to make an appointment.

Vitamins, Minerals, Fiber and Phytochemicals

Vitamins, minerals and fiber are all part of the nutrients we need every day. When we are talking about nutrients such vitamins and minerals, what do "good" and "excellent" sources mean? According to the Canadian Food Inspection Agency each vitamin and mineral has a Recommended Daily Intake (RDI) for both children under two and adults. Currently these are based on the 1983 Recommended Nutrient Intakes for Canadians (RNI), and represent the highest recommended intake of each nutrient for adults. These RNIs will soon be replaced by Dietary Reference Intakes (DRIs). Dietary Reference Intakes are a set of nutrient reference values for healthy populations that provide more detailed information on recommended nutrient levels including the Estimated Average Requirements (EAR) for most Canadians and the Tolerable Upper Intake Level (UL) which is the safe maximum recommended.

When a recipe indicates it is an excellent source of a particular nutrient this means that it contains greater than 25% of the RDI for that nutrient or equal to at least 50% in the case of vitamin C. Recipes high in certain nutrients are highlighted in the side bars of particular recipes and many are nutrient packed.

Remember that vitamins C, E and beta carotene (vitamin A) are thought to be antioxidant vitamins and may be protective against a number of diseases and potentially some of the complications of diabetes. Choosing foods high in these nutrients is a part of a healthy lifestyle.

Fiber, the indigestible portion of plant foods, is available as both soluble and insoluble. It is an important nutrient for a variety of reasons. Soluble fiber is found in fruits and vegetables, barley, legumes, oats, rye and seeds. When soluble fiber is consumed it slows the digestion of food and may help to control blood glucose rise after meals. Regular consumption of soluble fiber may help to lower cholesterol levels. Insoluble fiber, found in cereals, whole grains, beans and lentils, seeds and fruits and vegetables helps to promote regular elimination and may be helpful in reducing cancer risk. Choose high-fibre foods at every meal, where possible. On food labels, high-fiber foods are identified as those that contain 4 g or more of dietary fiber per serving. Very high fiber foods contain 6 g or more of dietary fiber per serving and those with 7 g or more can claim to "promote laxation" or "promote regularity." If you need more fiber, choose one of the many high-fiber recipes in this book.

Phytochemicals are substances found in plants which appear to have health benefits by helping to increase resistance against disease. They are found in a variety of different plants and have different effects on the human body. A few examples are carotenoids (such as beta carotene in carrots and lycopene in tomatoes), flavonoids (found in berries, celery, onions, grapes, soybeans, wholewheat products), lignans (part of the fiber found in flaxseed), phenolic acids (found in coffee beans, apples, blueberries, oranges, potatoes and soybeans and phytoesterols (found in soybeans and lentils).

When choosing to consume food sources of vitamins and minerals, you also obtain the benefit of fiber and phytochemicals. Thus, choosing to "eat" your vitamins and minerals offers benefits that no supplement can match.

Choosing to Sweeten

On average, "added sugars" contain 5 g of carbohydrate per teaspoon (5 mL), 0 g of protein, 0 g of fat and have an energy value of about 20 calories. (You will find the specific information listed on the nutrition panel on the label of these products.) The Canadian Diabetes Association suggests that added sugars can compose up to 10% of energy intake for a person with diabetes. What does that mean? In practical terms, if you are someone with an energy intake of about 1500 calories per day, about 150 could come from added sugars. This would equal about 7½ teaspoons (37 mL [38 g]) of added sugar per day. If your energy intake is about 2000 calories, then 200 calories or about 10 teaspoons (50 mL [50 g]) could come from added sugars.

When choosing to include "added sugars," keep in mind that many packaged products contain added sugar and this should be taken into consideration when choosing how much additional "added sugars" to include. For example, ketchup, salad dressings, creamed corn, coating mixes, cereals and many other items may contain sugar in a variety of forms. Use of products such these can quickly "use up" those "added sugars."

Remember that "added sugars" are a part of many recipes (including some in this book) in a variety of forms, including granulated white or brown sugar, corn syrup, honey, maple syrup or molasses. When these items are added to a recipe, the carbohydrate content is increased. For example, the recipe Quinoa Wraps with Hoisin Vegetables, page 70, contains 2 tbsp (25 mL) of honey, which contributes about 5 g of carbohydrate per serving

or about 1 tsp (5 mL) of "added sugar" per serving. By replacing the honey in this recipe with a granulated sugar substitute, you can reduce the carbohydrate content by about 5 g per serving and eliminate the ½ ✱ Sugars Choice. This may alter the taste slightly, but if you are trying to limit your carbohydrate intake at a meal, it is an easy way to keep within your target.

What should you choose?

That decision depends on several factors:

1. Your carbohydrate target for the meal. If you are trying to balance your intake by consuming a certain amount of carbohydrate or food choices from a meal plan, it may be beneficial to use a sugar substitute. If however, you can adjust your insulin or other food choices to account for the extra carbohydrate you may choose to leave in the added sugar.

2. Personal taste preference. You may wish to choose those products with "added sugars" over those containing sugar substitutes. If you prefer "added sugars," you may have to be more particular with your portion sizes to maintain your carbohydrate goals.

3. Change of recipe texture or results. In many cases, using a sugar substitute in products such as baked goods can alter the recipe texture, color and appearance. When using sugar substitutes be sure to follow the manufacturer's directions exactly for best results. Most companies have toll free information lines you can call for help.

Reducing Fat

On average, one teaspoon (5 mL) of fat contains 0 g of carbohydrate per teaspoon, 0 g of protein, 5 g of fat and has an energy value of about 45 calories. (You will find the specific information listed on the nutrition panel on the labels of these products.) It is recommended that fat contribute no more than 30% of energy intake for a person with diabetes, with less than 10% of energy intake from saturated fat.

In practical terms, if you are someone with an energy intake of about 1500 calories per day, about 450 could come from fat. This would equal about 10 teaspoons of fat (50 mL [50 g]) per day from all sources and of that, 3 teaspoons (15 mL [less than 15 g]) from saturated fat. If your energy intake is about 2000 calories, then 600 calories or about 13 teaspoons of fat (65 mL [65 g]) would supply about 30%. Saturated fat should supply less than 4 teaspoons (20 mL [20 g]) in a 2000 calorie diet.

Fat of various types is found in many foods. Fat is found in protein containing foods, milk products, dressings and sauces and added to many baked and prepared products. Check the product label to see how much fat is found in the product and choose the lower fat ones.

Most protein containing foods and milk products contain fat in the form of saturated fat. To limit your intake of saturated fat from these sources, try to:

- Choose lean cuts of meat and trim fat before cooking. Remove poultry skin and avoid food preparation methods such as deep frying, pan frying and those where fat is added.
- Avoid prepared packaged meats, such as deli meats and wieners, unless they are fat reduced.
- Choose low-fat dairy products, such as cheeses with a milk fat (M.F.) of 20% or less on the label.
- Choose low-fat milk such as 2%, 1% or skim.

Baked goods, prepared items and fast foods with hydrogenated vegetable oils or shortening, contain "trans fatty acids," which are similar to saturated fat and have the same effect on blood lipid (cholesterol) levels. Try to avoid products containing hydrogenated vegetable oils and shortening by:

- Choosing baked goods prepared with soft margarine or vegetable oils such as canola, olive or peanut oil.
- Looking at the labels for products, which contain less than 1 teaspoon (5 mL [5 g]) of fat per serving).
- Preparing your own baked goods at home.

When using fat, try to keep the following in mind:

- Choose oils such as canola, olive or peanut oil.
- Choose an non-hydrogenated unsaturated margarine in a soft tub where the polyunsaturated and monounsaturated fats listed on the label are at least 75% of the total fat.
- If you have added fat during cooking, limit the amount of fat you include at the table.
- Nuts and seeds contain unsaturated fat, but are very high in energy. Enjoy them sparingly if you are trying to manage your weight.
- Remember that all fats supply an equal amount of energy; so even if the fat is unsaturated, it is wise to limit its use. This is particularly important if you are trying to lose or maintain your weight.

Good Health Eating Guide System

The Good Health Eating Guide system of meal planning is a system known to many individuals with diabetes throughout Canada. Based on *Canada's Food Guide* and *Canada's Guidelines for Healthy Eating*, it translates the information into practical meal planning choices for people with diabetes. The Good Health Eating Guide provides information on a variety of foods by classifying those containing similar macronutrients (carbohydrate, protein, fat and energy [calories]) into one of the seven Food Choice groups shown below:

■ Starch Foods

Starch foods all contribute to a rise in blood glucose and are a key part of a diabetes meal plan. Some choices contain dietary fiber, either as soluble, insoluble or in combination, both of which play important roles in good health and diabetes meal planning.

One choice contains about 15 g carbohydrate, 2 g protein, 0 g fat, and has a 290 kJ (68 calories) energy value.

Examples of one ■ Starch Choice are:
1 slice (30 g) wholegrain bread
⅓ cup (75 mL) of rice
½ cup (125 mL) cooked barley
½ cup (125 mL) cooked beans or lentils
½ cup (125 mL) cooked cereal
½ English muffin
6 soda crackers
½ hamburger or hot dog bun
1 shredded wheat
2 rice cakes
½ cup (125 mL) cooked pasta
1 small plain roll

■ Fruits & Vegetables

All fruits, all juices and some vegetables contain carbohydrate as naturally occurring sugar. They are an important source of vitamins and minerals in the diet and all raise blood glucose levels.

One choice contains about 10 g carbohydrate, 1 g protein, 0 g fat, and has a 190 kJ (44 calories) energy value.

Examples of one ■ Fruits & Vegetables Choice are:
½ medium apple
2 apricots
½ small banana
½ cup (125 mL) grapes
¼ cantaloupe
½ cup (125 mL) cut up fresh fruit
10 cherries
½ grapefruit
½ cup (125 mL) fresh beets
½ cup (125 mL) carrots
½ cup (125 mL) squash
½ cup (125 mL) mixed vegetables

◆ Milk

All forms of milk contain carbohydrate as lactose, the naturally occurring sugar in milk. Milk is an important source of calcium in the diet of many Canadians and also provides other vitamins and minerals like vitamin D, phosphorus and riboflavin.

One choice contains about 6 g carbohydrate, 4 g protein, 0 to 4 g fat, and has a 170 kJ (40 calories) to 320 kJ (76 calories) energy value depending upon the type of milk.

Examples of one ◆ Milk Choice are:
½ cup (125 mL) milk
½ cup (125 mL) of buttermilk
¼ cup (50 mL) evaporated milk
½ cup (125 mL) plain yogurt

✱ Sugars

The Sugars group contains foods with added sugar from a variety of sources, which are also a part of meal planning for diabetes. As with all other foods containing carbohydrate, they contribute to a rise in blood glucose. Nutrition guidelines suggest that added sugars can comprise up to 10% of the total daily energy in the diet of people with diabetes. Added sugars contribute little in the way of nutrients to meal planning, but when substituted for other carbohydrates they increase meal plan flexibility and choice.

One choice contains about 10 g of carbohydrate, 0 g of protein, and 0 g of fat and has 168 kJ (40 calories) energy value.

Examples of one ✱ Sugars Choice are:
2 tsp (10 mL) white or brown sugar
1 tbsp (15 mL) regular jam, jelly or
    marmalade
2 small sweet pickles
2 tbsp (25 mL) sweet relish
2 hard candies
4 jelly beans
½ popsicle
2 large marshmallows
1 piece of bubble gum
⅓ cup (75 mL) regular cranberry cocktail
2 tsp (10 mL) honey, molasses, maple
    or corn syrup
½ cup (125 mL) regular soft drink

◉ Protein Foods

Protein Foods are made up of choices like fish, lean meat, poultry, cheese and those from plant sources such as peanut butter, soybeans, tofu and lentils. Most protein foods do not contain carbohydrate and do not directly affect blood glucose levels. In addition to providing protein, many of the animal forms contain minerals such as iron and fats such as omega-3 fatty acids while the vegetable forms may contain plant sterols and phytochemicals.

One choice usually contains about 0 g carbohydrate, 7 g protein, 3 g fat, and has a 230 kJ (55 calories) energy value.

Examples of one ◉ Protein Choice are:
1 oz (30 g) fish
¼ cup (50 mL) canned salmon
3 medium clams, mussels, scallops
5 large shrimp
1 slice (1 oz/30 g) lean meat or chicken
1 medium egg
1 slice low-fat (7% m.f.) cheese
¼ cup (50 mL) 2% cottage cheese
½ block (70 g) tofu
½ chop (40 g), with bone
2 tbsp (25 mL) lean ground chicken
    or beef
1 slice (30 g) heart or liver

▲ Fats & Oils

Fats and oils add energy to the diet and some provide a source of essential fatty acids. While fats contribute energy to the diet, it is very important for people with diabetes to watch both the amount of fat and type of fat they choose. Monounsaturated fats found in some plant oils (canola, olive and peanut) are the preferred choice. Both saturated and polyunsaturated fats should be limited to no more than 10% of energy intake or the equivalent of about 4 to 5 ▲ Fats & Oils Choices (or teaspoons) per day.

One choice contains about 0 g protein, 5 g fat, 0 g carbohydrate and has a 190 kJ (45 calories) energy value.

Examples of one ▲ Fats & Oils Choice are:

1 tsp (5 mL) oil
10 peanuts
1 tsp (5 mL) margarine
1 tbsp (15 mL) sunflower seeds (shelled)
2 tbsp (25 mL) low-calorie salad dressing
5 tsp (25 mL) pine nuts
1 tbsp (15 mL) cheese spread
7 black olives
1 slice bacon, side crisp*
1 tbsp (15 mL) dried unsweetened
   coconut*
1 tbsp (15 mL) whipping cream*
2 tbsp (25 mL) sour cream (12% m.f.)*
* These items are sources of saturated fat.

✽✽ Extras

The Extras add variety to diabetes meal planning. The foods in this group include both vegetables and other items, which are both low in calories and carbohydrate. The Extra vegetables in this section can provide valuable vitamins, minerals and phytochemicals in the meal plan of someone with diabetes. As most of these vegetables are low in carbohydrate, when eaten in small quantities, they do not have to be counted in your meal plan.

One choice usually contains less than 2.5 g carbohydrate, 0 g protein, 0 g fat, and has a 60 kJ (15 calories) energy.

Examples of one ✽✽ Extra Choice are:

Extra Vegetables
Artichokes
Asparagus
Broccoli
Cabbage
Cauliflower
Cucumber
Lettuce
Mushrooms
Peppers, green, red and yellow
Spinach

Extras
Coffee
Flavorings and Extracts
Garlic
Lemon juice
Mineral water
Sugar-free gelatin desserts
Sugar-free soft drinks
Tea
Vinegar
Spices

The Good Health Eating Guide system is composed of both a poster and resource book. These are available from:
- Your health care team at your local diabetes center;
- A dietitian at your local hospital or community health centre;
- The provincial branch or national office of the Canadian Diabetes Association.

Carbohydrate Counting

Carbohydrate counting is one method of meal management used by people with diabetes as an alternative to following a meal plan. People choosing to carbohydrate count are often those people who use a rapid acting insulin, which they can adjust depending on their carbohydrate consumption. Those with type 2 diabetes managed by meal planning (with or without oral diabetes medication) may use this method to aim for carbohydrate targets at meals. This method increases flexibility in meal planning for many people.

What are the principles of carbohydrate counting?

Carbohydrate found in foods is known to be the primary source of glucose in the blood.

Although both of the other "macronutrients," protein and fat, can be broken down into carbohydrate, this will not usually occur, except when there is inadequate carbohydrate available to the body for energy.

There are several forms of carbohydrate, some which contribute to blood glucose and some which do not. These are sugars, starch, dietary fiber and "sugar alcohols." The latter are usually seen in products developed for people with diabetes such as "no sugar added" candies; small amounts sometimes occur naturally in foods.

Dietary fiber, primarily undigested by the body, is one of the components of carbohydrate which does not raise the blood glucose. Therefore when counting carbohydrate, *it is important to remove the dietary fiber from the total carbohydrate* to determine the available carbohydrate. **Available carbohydrate is the carbohydrate which will contribute to a rise in blood glucose.**

Are there concerns with carbohydrate counting?

People who choose to carbohydrate count should always keep good nutrition in mind. With increased meal flexibility, some food choices incorporated may provide less nutrition. For example, if choosing to eat high fat, high carbohydrate desserts regularly, these may take the place of more nutritious choices such as fresh fruit with meals. What are the consequences of this? For those using insulin, larger amounts of rapid acting insulin may be required to achieve blood glucose targets and over time this may lead to weight gain. Making these choices can also impact on weight and blood fat (cholesterol) levels. Lastly, substituting low-nutrient foods for healthier selections may deprive the body of a number of essential nutrients such as calcium, vitamins A and C, fiber and a whole host of others.

Working with a dietitian

Work with the dietitian from your diabetes health care team if you are thinking about using carbohydrate counting as a method of meal planning. Together you can review the essentials of carbohydrate counting, look at your regular intake to determine an appropriate carbohydrate/insulin ratio and work through any difficulties that result when you begin.

Those choosing to carbohydrate count learn to adjust their meal intake to meet their individual targets or if using insulin, may adjust their dose to cover their carbohydrate intake. If you plan your meals and snacks by counting carbohydrate, there are two ways to do this:

METHOD 1

Use the Canadian Diabetes Association Food Choice Values and Symbols system. With this method, all the nutrient information affecting the available carbohydrate has been considered before determining the Food Choice Values and Symbols.

Carbohydrate is found in four of the seven food choice groups on the Good Health Eating Guide. Here is the amount of carbohydrate in 1 Food Choice in each of the seven Food Choice groups.

Food Choices	Grams of Carbohydrates
1 ■ Starch	15
1 ◗ Fruits & Vegetables	10
1 ◆ Milk	6
1 ✳ Sugars	10
1 ◕ Protein	0
1 ▲ Fats & Oils	0
1 ✦✦ Extras	0

If you are using a recipe such as Tex-Mex Pork Chops with Black Bean Salsa, page 93, where the Food Choice Value listed is 2 ■ + ½ ◗ + 4 ◕ , you can determine the available carbohydrate by looking at the Food Choices for each and multiply the grams of carbohydrate per food group, then add them together to obtain a total.

Food Choice	Grams of carbohydrate per choice		Available carbohydrate
2 ■ x	15	=	30 g
½ ◗ x	10	=	5 g
4 ◕ x	0	=	0 g
Available carbohydrate		=	35 g

METHOD 2

You may also count carbohydrate by looking at the nutrient information listed on recipes or product labels. Simply take the amount of carbohydrate listed and subtract the fiber. This provides you with the amount of "available" carbohydrate per recipe.

For example, on page 93 the nutrition information for the Tex-Mex Pork Chops with Black Bean Salsa recipe indicates:

Calories	400 kcal
Carbohydrate	45 g
Fiber	12 g
Protein	35 g
Fat, total	10 g
Fat, saturated	2 g
Sodium	218 mg
Cholesterol	51 mg

Carbohydrate 45 g – Fiber 12 g = Available Carbohydrate 33 g

The small difference in grams of carbohydrate using these two methods is within the "tolerance" allowed for carbohydrate counting.

Using this information together with the carbohydrate from the other foods in your meal you can estimate the total amount of available carbohydrate and determine how much insulin to take based on your carbohydrate to insulin ratio. It is important to work with the dietitian on your diabetes health care team to determine your individual carbohydrate to insulin ratio and to become comfortable with this method of meal planning. Keep healthy eating and good nutrition in mind.

Glycemic Index

The "glycemic index" is a scale which ranks carbohydrate rich foods by how much they raise blood glucose levels compared to a standard food. After eating carbohydrate containing foods, blood glucose levels rise and the extent of that rise is called the "glycemic response." The "glycemic index" of different foods has been compared to a standard "glucose" response and the effect of these foods on blood glucose has been given a value. (See table right.)

There are many factors which contribute to a food's glycemic effect and this may be due in part to the soluble fiber contained in the food, how resistant the carbohydrate containing food is to digestion, how the food has been cooked or prepared and whether the food is eaten alone or as part of a mixed meal.

For people with diabetes, this means that by choosing foods that have a low glycemic index more often, there may be less of a rise in blood glucose after meals or snacks. In some instances, where people have regularly chosen low glycemic index foods, they have required less insulin. Other benefits of choosing low glycemic index foods include making food choices which are often higher in vitamins, minerals and fiber and increased satiety. There is also some research indicating that people at risk for diabetes may reduce their risk by regularly choosing foods which have a low glycemic index.

More information on the glycemic index can be found on the Canadian Diabetes Association website: www.diabetes.ca.

Glycemic Index Exchanges

Lowest Glycemic Index to High Glycemic Index

Pearl barley	25
Legumes	25-48
Tomato soup	38
Spaghetti	41
Parboiled rice	47
Bran Buds with Psyllium®	47
Bulgur (cracked wheat)	48
Red River Cereal®	49
Chocolate	49
Rye kernel-pumpernickel bread	50
Yams	51
Oat Bran	55
Polished rice	56
Pita Bread	57
Oatmeal	61
White/ whole/ canned potatoes	61
Boxed macaroni and cheese	64
Rye crisp bread	65
Couscous	65
Shredded wheat	69
Whole wheat bread	69
White wheat bread	70
Cornmeal	70
Mashed potato	70-83
Corn chips	73
Puffed Wheat®	74
French fries	75
Jelly beans	80
Cornflakes®	84
Puffed Rice®	86
Rice cakes	88
Glucose	100

References: Wolever, T.M.S., Glycemic Index Workshop, 2000.

Recipe Analysis

The recipes were analyzed using the Nutriwatch Nutrient Analysis Program (Canadian Nutrient file 2000), Version 6.120E, Delphi 1, copyright 2000, Elizabeth Warwick. Where necessary additional data was supplemented using the USDA database on line.

Analysis information was based on:

- Imperial measures and weights were used, except where metric measurements were listed.
- The larger number of servings was used when there was a range.
- The first ingredient and amount were used where alternatives were specified.
- Optional ingredients were not included.
- Calculations including meat and poultry used lean portions without skin.
- Soft margarine and canola oil were used in recipe analysis where the type of fat was not specified.

The milk and cheese listed for the specific recipe has been used in the analysis, however in most instances, if not already low fat, you should be able to successfully use lower-fat milk and low-fat cheese to further reduce the fat content.

Nutrient values were rounded to the nearest whole number for presentation in the text. In calculation of the Canadian Diabetes Association Food Choice Values, the actual nutrient values were used, prior to rounding.

Editor's note: No sugar added yogurt is suggested in side bars to complete a number of meals. Your personal carbohydrate targets for a meal may permit you to use a regular yogurt instead.

Starters
and Salads

Melizzano Despina (Eggplant Dip)

Tips

It works wonderfully as a smoky-oniony dip for raw vegetables and also as a spread on sandwiches.

This dip can be served immediately or it can wait, covered and unrefrigerated, for up to 2 hours. If refrigerated, let it come back to room temperature and give it a couple of stirs before serving.

1	medium eggplant (about 1 lb/500 g)	1
1 tsp	vegetable oil	5 mL
1	onion	1
2 tbsp	lemon juice	25 mL
¼ cup	olive oil	50 mL
	Few sprigs fresh parsley, chopped	
	Salt and pepper to taste	

1. Brush eggplant lightly with vegetable oil. Using a fork, pierce the skin lightly at 1-inch (2.5-cm) intervals. Place on a baking sheet and bake for 1 hour, or until eggplant is very soft and the skin is dark brown and caved in.

2. Transfer eggplant to a working surface. Cut off 1 inch (2 cm) at the stem end and discard (this part never quite cooks through). Peel the eggplant by picking at an edge from the cut end, then pulling upward. The skin should come off easily in strips.

3. Cut the eggplant lengthwise and place each half with the interior facing you. With a spoon scoop out the tongues of seed-pods, leaving as much of the flesh as possible. To remove the additional seed-pods hiding inside, cut each piece of eggplant in half and repeat the deseeding procedure. Once deseeded, let cleaned eggplant flesh sit to shed some of its excess water.

continued on page 21

NUTRIENT ANALYSIS PER SERVING			
Calories	166	Fat, total	15 g
Carbohydrates	9 g	Fat, saturated	2 g
Fiber	0 g	Sodium	4 mg
Protein	1 g	Cholesterol	0 mg

4. Transfer drained eggplant flesh to a bowl. Using a wooden spoon, mash and then whip the pulp until smooth and very soft. Coarsely grate onion directly into the eggplant (the onion juice that results is very important to this dip). Add lemon juice and whip with a wooden spoon until perfectly integrated. Keep beating and add olive oil in a very thin stream; the result should be a frothy, light colored emulsion. Season to taste with salt and pepper. Transfer to a serving bowl and garnish with chopped parsley.

Rosy Shrimp Spread

Tips

Microwave cold cream cheese at Medium for 1 minute to soften.

This spread is equally good with crackers or vegetable dippers.

Instead of shrimp, try using 1 can (6 oz/170 g) crab.

Make Ahead

Spread can be prepared up to 2 days ahead, covered and refrigerated.

4 oz	light cream cheese, softened	125 g
¼ cup	light sour cream or plain yogurt	50 mL
2 tbsp	prepared chili sauce	25 mL
1 tsp	prepared horseradish	5 mL
	Hot pepper sauce, to taste	
1	can (4 oz/113 g) small shrimp, rinsed and drained	1
1 tbsp	minced green onion tops or chives	15 mL

1. In a bowl, beat cream cheese until smooth. Stir in sour cream, chili sauce, horseradish and hot pepper sauce.

2. Fold in shrimp and green onions. Transfer to serving dish; cover and refrigerate until serving time.

FOOD CHOICE VALUES PER ¹⁄₁₀ OF RECIPE (2 TBSP/25 ML)

½ ◨ Protein Choice

NUTRIENT ANALYSIS PER SERVING			
Calories	48	Fat, total	3 g
Carbohydrates	2 g	Fat, saturated	1 g
Fiber	0 g	Sodium	127 mg
Protein	4 g	Cholesterol	27 mg

This is a lovely
summer party dish.

To make this a
complete meal, serve
with whole grain bread,
milk and low-fat cheese.

Avocado Melissa Sue Anderson

2 tbsp	lime juice	25 mL
2	ripe avocados	2
1	Granny Smith apple, peeled and thinly sliced	1
2	peaches, peeled and cut into chunks	2
5	green onions, cut into ½-inch (1-cm) pieces	5
3 cups	sliced mushrooms	750 mL
2	stalks celery, chopped	2
¾ cup	unpeeled, diced English cucumber	175 mL
2	tomatoes, cubed	2
⅓ cup	toasted cashew pieces	75 mL
3 tbsp	finely chopped fresh coriander	45 mL
2 tbsp	vegetable oil	25 mL
1 tbsp	sesame oil	15 mL
1 tbsp	raspberry (or white wine) vinegar	15 mL
1 tsp	salt	5 mL
1 tsp	cayenne (optional)	5 mL
	Alfalfa sprouts	

1. Put lime juice in a large bowl. Peel avocado and cut into slices (or scoop out with a small spoon) and add to the lime juice. Toss gently until well coated. Add apple slices and toss again. Add peaches, green onions, mushrooms, celery, cucumber, tomato and cashew pieces.

2. In a small bowl whisk together coriander, vegetable oil, sesame oil, vinegar, salt and optional cayenne until emulsified. Drizzle half of the dressing over the salad. Fold in the dressing, mixing the various ingredients of the salad. Do this gently but thoroughly. Add the rest of the dressing, and fold in 5 or 6 more times.

continued on page 23

FOOD CHOICE VALUES PER SERVING

1 🥬 Fruit & Vegetable Choice

2½ ▲ Fats & Oils Choices

NUTRIENT ANALYSIS PER SERVING			
Calories	159	Fat, total	13 g
Carbohydrates	12 g	Fat, saturated	2 g
Fiber	3 g	Sodium	276 mg
Protein	3 g	Cholesterol	0 mg

3. Transfer to a serving bowl and garnish with alfalfa sprouts for that final California touch. Serve immediately or keep up to 1 hour, covered and unrefrigerated.

Pico De Gallo (Mexican Hot Sauce)

MAKES ABOUT 1 CUP (250 ML)

Tips

This delicious, versatile and explosive sauce requires no cooking, and can live in the fridge nicely for 2 to 3 days, though it is best about an hour after it's freshly made. The hotness of the sauce can be regulated by modifying the amount of jalapeno pepper seeds used.

When working with hot peppers, be sure to wear gloves; otherwise, wash hands thoroughly.

1	medium tomato, cut into 1/4-inch (0.5-cm) cubes	1
1/4 cup	finely diced red onions	50 mL
2	jalapeno peppers, finely diced (with or without seeds, depending on desired hotness)	2
1/2 tsp	salt	2 mL
1 tbsp	lime juice	15 mL
1 tbsp	vegetable oil	15 mL
	Few sprigs fresh coriander, chopped	

1. In bowl combine tomato, onions, jalapeno, salt and lime juice. Stir to mix well. Add oil and stir again.

2. Transfer to a serving bowl and scatter chopped coriander on top. Let rest for about 1 hour, covered and unrefrigerated, for best flavor. Serve alongside main courses and appetizers.

FOOD CHOICE VALUES PER 1/4 OF RECIPE (1/4 CUP/60 ML)

1/2 ◨ Fruit & Vegetable Choice

1/2 ▲ Fats & Oils Choice

NUTRIENT ANALYSIS PER SERVING			
Calories	44	Fat, total	4 g
Carbohydrates	3 g	Fat, saturated	0 g
Fiber	1 g	Sodium	365 mg
Protein	1 g	Cholesterol	0 mg

Tips

Wheat berries are unprocessed whole kernels of wheat. They're tender, chewy and crunchy — great for salads and pilafs! Wheat berries are also extremely nutritious, and make a great high-fiber substitute in traditional meat loaf recipes.

This recipe is an excellent source of vitamins A and C.

Wheat Berry Salad with Sesame Dressing

DRESSING

1 tbsp	honey	15 mL
1 tbsp	rice wine vinegar	15 mL
1 tbsp	sesame oil	15 mL
1 tbsp	toasted sesame seeds	15 mL
1 tbsp	light soya sauce	15 mL
1 tbsp	tahini (sesame paste)	15 mL
1 tsp	minced garlic	5 mL
½ tsp	minced gingerroot	2 mL

SALAD

3½ cups	seafood stock or chicken stock	875 mL
1 cup	wheat berries	250 mL
½ cup	thinly sliced green onions	125 mL
½ cup	diced carrots	125 mL
½ cup	diced green bell peppers	125 mL
½ cup	diced red bell peppers	125 mL
½ cup	diced snow peas	125 mL
8 oz	scallops	250 g

1. *Dressing:* In a bowl combine honey, rice wine vinegar, sesame oil, sesame seeds, soya sauce, tahini, garlic and ginger; whisk well. Set aside.

2. *Salad:* In a saucepan over high heat, bring stock to a boil. Add wheat berries; reduce heat to low. Cook, covered, for approximately 45 minutes or until berries are tender but chewy. Drain any excess liquid; allow to cool. Add green onions, carrots, green peppers, red peppers and snow peas. Set aside.

3. In a nonstick frying pan sprayed with vegetable spray or on a preheated grill, cook scallops over medium-high heat for 3 minutes or until cooked through. Drain any excess liquid; dice scallops.

continued on page 25

FOOD CHOICE VALUES PER SERVING

1	■	Starch Choice
1	◗	Fruit & Vegetable Choice
½	✳	Sugars Choice
1½	◓	Protein Choices

NUTRIENT ANALYSIS PER SERVING

Calories	225	Fat, total	6 g
Carbohydrates	31 g	Fat, saturated	1 g
Fiber	2 g	Sodium	366 mg
Protein	14 g	Cholesterol	19 mg

4. In a serving bowl, combine wheat berry mixture, scallops and dressing; toss to coat well. Serve.

SERVES 6

Tips
Here's a great twist on traditional coleslaw, with the sweet flavors of apricots, fennel and balsamic vinegar.

Toast nuts in a nonstick skillet over high heat until browned, about 2 to 3 minutes.

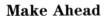

Make Ahead
Prepare up to 1 day in advance. Best if tossed just before serving.

Red-and-Green Coleslaw with Apricots and Fennel

SALAD

3 cups	thinly sliced green cabbage	750 mL
3 cups	thinly sliced red cabbage	750 mL
1 1/2 cups	thinly sliced red bell peppers	375 mL
1 cup	chopped dried apricots	250 mL
1 cup	canned corn kernels, drained	250 mL
1 cup	thinly sliced fennel	250 mL
1/2 cup	chopped green onions	125 mL
1/4 cup	toasted slivered almonds	50 mL
2 tbsp	toasted sesame seeds	25 mL

DRESSING

1/4 cup	balsamic vinegar	50 mL
3 tbsp	olive oil	45 mL
1 1/2 tsp	minced garlic	7 mL

1. *Salad:* In a large bowl, combine green cabbage, red cabbage, red peppers, apricots, corn, fennel, green onions, almonds and sesame seeds.

2. *Dressing:* In a small bowl, whisk together vinegar, oil and garlic.

3. Pour dressing over salad; toss to coat.

FOOD CHOICE VALUES PER SERVING

2 1/2 ◖ Fruit & Vegetable Choices

1/2 ◕ Protein Choice

2 ▲ Fats & Oils Choices

NUTRIENT ANALYSIS PER SERVING

Calories	224	Fat, total	12 g
Carbohydrates	30 g	Fat, saturated	2 g
Fiber	5 g	Sodium	107 mg
Protein	5 g	Cholesterol	0 mg

Tips
The vegetables and
dried fruit give this salad
a wonderful flavor
and texture.

Substitute coriander,
basil or parsley for
the dill.

This recipe is an
excellent source
of vitamins A and C
and folic acid.

Make Ahead
Prepare early in the day.
Best served chilled.

Broccoli, Apricot and Red Pepper Salad in a Creamy Dressing

4 cups	broccoli florets	1 L
1 cup	chopped carrots	250 mL
1 cup	sliced red bell peppers	250 mL
¾ cup	sliced water chestnuts	175 mL
½ cup	chopped red onions	125 mL
½ cup	chopped dried apricots or dates	125 mL
⅓ cup	raisins	75 mL
2 oz	feta cheese, crumbled	50 g

DRESSING

¼ cup	chopped fresh dill	50 mL
¼ cup	light mayonnaise	50 mL
¼ cup	light sour cream	50 mL
2 tbsp	freshly squeezed lemon juice	25 mL
1 ½ tsp	minced garlic	7 mL
	Freshly ground black pepper, to taste	

1. Boil or steam broccoli 3 minutes or until tender-crisp; drain. Rinse under cold water; drain well.

2. In a large serving bowl, combine broccoli, carrots, red peppers, water chestnuts, red onions, apricots, raisins and feta cheese.

3. *Dressing:* In a small bowl, whisk together dill, mayonnaise, sour cream, lemon juice and garlic. Pour over salad; toss to coat. Season to taste with pepper.

FOOD CHOICE VALUES PER SERVING

2½ ◖ Fruit & Vegetable Choices

½ ◙ Protein Choice

1 ▲ Fats & Oils Choice

NUTRIENT ANALYSIS PER SERVING			
Calories	181	Fat, total	6 g
Carbohydrates	31 g	Fat, saturated	2 g
Fiber	5 g	Sodium	208 mg
Protein	5 g	Cholesterol	9 mg

Soups and
Sandwiches

Vegetable Stock

Tip
Here's the perfect
stock for vegetarians.
It keeps for up to
6 months if frozen in
airtight containers.

6 cups	water	1.5 L
1	large sweet potato, diced	1
2	large celery stalks, chopped	2
2	large leeks, cleaned and sliced	2
1	large onion, chopped	1
1/2 cup	chopped parsley	125 mL
2	large cloves garlic	2
2	bay leaves	2
1/4 tsp	freshly ground black pepper	1 mL
1/8 tsp	salt	0.5 mL

1. In a saucepan over medium-high heat, combine water, potato, celery, leeks, onion, parsley, garlic, bay leaves, pepper and salt; bring to a boil. Reduce heat to low; simmer, covered, for 1½ hours.

2. Pour mixture through a strainer; discard solids. Refrigerate stock until cold. Stock can be kept, refrigerated, for up to 3 days or frozen in an airtight container.

NUTRIENT ANALYSIS PER SERVING

Calories	8	Fat, total	0 g
Carbohydrates	2 g	Fat, saturated	0 g
Fiber	0 g	Sodium	47 mg
Protein	0 g	Cholesterol	0 mg

Fish Stock

6 cups	water	1.5 L
1½ lbs	fish or seafood pieces	750 g
1	large carrot, peeled and chopped	1
1	medium onion, quartered	1
1	large celery stalk, chopped	1
3	large cloves garlic	3
¼ tsp	freshly ground black pepper	1 mL
⅛ tsp	salt	0.5 mL
½ cup	chopped parsley	125 mL
2	bay leaves	2

1. In a saucepan over medium-high heat, combine water, fish/seafood pieces, carrot, onion, celery, garlic, pepper, salt, parsley, and bay leaves. Bring to a boil, skimming any foam that rises to the top. cover, reduce heat to low; simmer for 1½ hours.

2. Pour mixture through a strainer; discard solids. Refrigerate stock until cold; skim fat off surface. Stock can be refrigerated for up to 3 days or frozen in an airtight container.

FOOD CHOICE VALUES PER ⅙ OF RECIPE

1 ✦✦ Extra Choice

NUTRIENT ANALYSIS PER SERVING			
Calories	13	Fat, total	0 g
Carbohydrates	1 g	Fat, saturated	0 g
Fiber	0 g	Sodium	54 mg
Protein	2 g	Cholesterol	6 mg

Sun-Dried Tomato Pesto is optional, but it adds a wonderful jolt of flavor and dresses up the soup. You can also use whatever pesto you have on hand.

Serve with additional Parmesan cheese at the table. Refrigerate soup for up to five days or freeze in airtight containers for up to three months.

Rinse the canned Romano beans thoroughly to further reduce the sodium in this recipe.

If you don't have time to make the vegetable stock on page 28, using a low-sodium chicken stock will increase sodium to 827 mg. Regular stock increases sodium to 1971 mg per serving.

The vegetables in this soup makes it an excellent source of vitamin A.

Vegetable Minestrone with Sun-Dried Tomato Pesto

1 tbsp	olive oil	15 mL
2	large onions, chopped	2
3	cloves garlic, finely chopped	3
2	carrots, peeled and chopped	2
2	stalks celery, chopped	2
10 cups	vegetable stock (see recipe, page 28) or low-sodium chicken stock (approx.)	2.5 L
2 cups	shredded cabbage	500 mL
2 cups	small cauliflower florets	500 mL
1/3 cup	short fine noodles or other small-shaped pasta such as shells	75 mL
1 cup	frozen peas	250 mL
1	can (19 oz/540 mL) Romano or navy beans, drained and rinsed	1
3/4 cup	Sun-Dried Tomato Pesto (see recipe, following)	175 mL
	Freshly grated Parmesan cheese (optional)	

1. In a large stockpot or 32-cup (8 L) Dutch oven, heat oil over medium heat. Add onions, garlic, carrots and celery; cook, stirring occasionally, for 10 minutes or until softened.

2. Add stock and cabbage; bring to a boil over high heat. Reduce heat, cover and simmer for 20 minutes or just until vegetables are tender. Stir in cauliflower and pasta; simmer, covered, for 8 minutes or just until pasta is tender. Stir in peas and beans; cook for 2 minutes.

3. Ladle into bowls; swirl a generous tablespoon (15 mL) Sun-Dried Tomato Pesto into each. Sprinkle with Parmesan cheese, if desired. Soup thickens slightly as it cools; add more stock, if necessary.

FOOD CHOICE VALUES PER SERVING

1½ ◖ Fruit & Vegetable Choices

1 ◑ Protein Choice

1 ▲ Fats & Oils Choice

NUTRIENT ANALYSIS PER SERVING

Calories	167	Fat, total	8 g
Carbohydrates	18 g	Fat, saturated	2 g
Fiber	3 g	Sodium	265 mg
Protein	7 g	Cholesterol	3 mg

Sun-Dried Tomato Pesto

½ cup	sun-dried tomatoes	125 mL
½ cup	lightly packed fresh basil	125 mL
½ cup	lightly packed fresh parsley	125 mL
1	large clove garlic	1
⅓ cup	vegetable stock (see recipe, page 28)	75 mL
2 tbsp	olive oil	25 mL
⅓ cup	freshly grated Parmesan cheese	75 mL
½ tsp	freshly ground black pepper	2 mL

1. In a bowl, cover sun-dried tomatoes with boiling water; let stand for 10 minutes or until softened. Drain and pat dry; chop coarsely.

2. In a food processor, combine rehydrated tomatoes, basil, parsley and garlic. With motor running, add stock and oil in a stream. Stir in Parmesan cheese and pepper.

Tip

For a fast dinner suggestion, toss this pesto with cooked pasta. (Remember, ½ cup/125 mL cooked pasta equals 1 ■ Starch Choice.) Complete the meal with low-fat, no sugar added yogurt over fruit if your meal plan permits.

FOOD CHOICE VALUES PER ⅓ OF RECIPE

1	◗	Fruit & Vegetable Choice
1	◑	Protein Choice
2	▲	Fats & Oils Choices

NUTRIENT ANALYSIS PER SERVING

Calories	170	Fat, total	13 g
Carbohydrates	8 g	Fat, saturated	3 g
Fiber	0 g	Sodium	465 mg
Protein	7 g	Cholesterol	9 mg

Tip

If you have to watch your salt intake, keep in mind that store-bought canned bouillon, powder and cubed stocks are high in sodium. Making your own stock is a much healthier alternative. Take a look at the stock recipes on pages 28–29 and give them a try. For chicken and beef stocks, refrigerate overnight, remove any layers of fat and freeze in containers for later use.

Barley Minestrone with Pesto

1 cup	chopped onions	250 mL
1 1/2 tsp	minced garlic	7 mL
1 1/2 cups	diced unpeeled zucchini	375 mL
1 cup	diced unpeeled eggplant	250 mL
1/2 cup	diced carrots	125 mL
4 3/4 cups	vegetable stock (see recipe, page 28) or chicken stock	1.175 L
1	can (19 oz/540 mL) whole tomatoes, with juice	1
1 1/2 cups	diced peeled potatoes	375 mL
1 cup	canned cooked white kidney beans, rinsed and drained	250 mL
1/3 cup	pearl barley	75 mL
2 1/2 tsp	dried basil	12 mL
1	bay leaf	1
2 tbsp	pesto	25 mL
3 tbsp	grated low-fat Parmesan cheese	45 mL

1. In a large nonstick saucepan sprayed with vegetable spray, cook onions and garlic over medium-high heat for 2 minutes or until softened. Add zucchini, eggplant and carrots; cook for 5 minutes, stirring occasionally.

2. Add stock, tomatoes (with juice), potatoes, kidney beans, barley, basil and bay leaf. Bring to a boil, breaking tomatoes with back of a spoon. Reduce heat to medium-low; cook, covered, for 45 minutes or until barley is tender.

3. Ladle soup into bowls. Spoon a dollop of pesto in center of each serving; garnish with Parmesan cheese.

FOOD CHOICE VALUES PER SERVING

1 ■ Starch Choice

1/2 ◢ Fruit & Vegetable Choice

1/2 ◢ Protein Choice

NUTRIENT ANALYSIS PER SERVING

Calories	135	Fat, total	1 g
Carbohydrates	28 g	Fat, saturated	0 g
Fiber	5 g	Sodium	306 mg
Protein	5 g	Cholesterol	0 mg

Vegetable Minestrone with Sun-Dried Tomato Pesto (page 30)

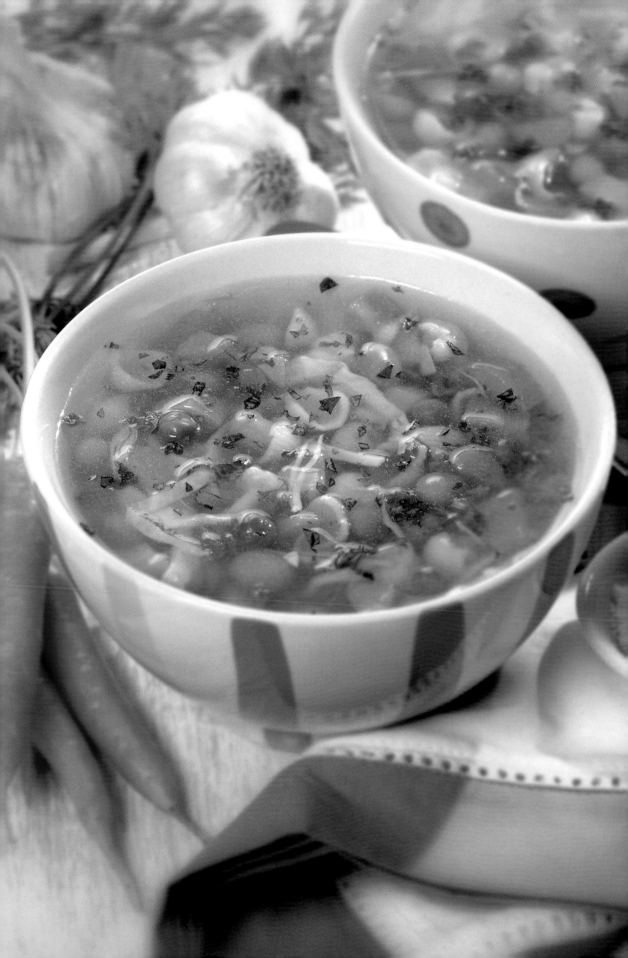

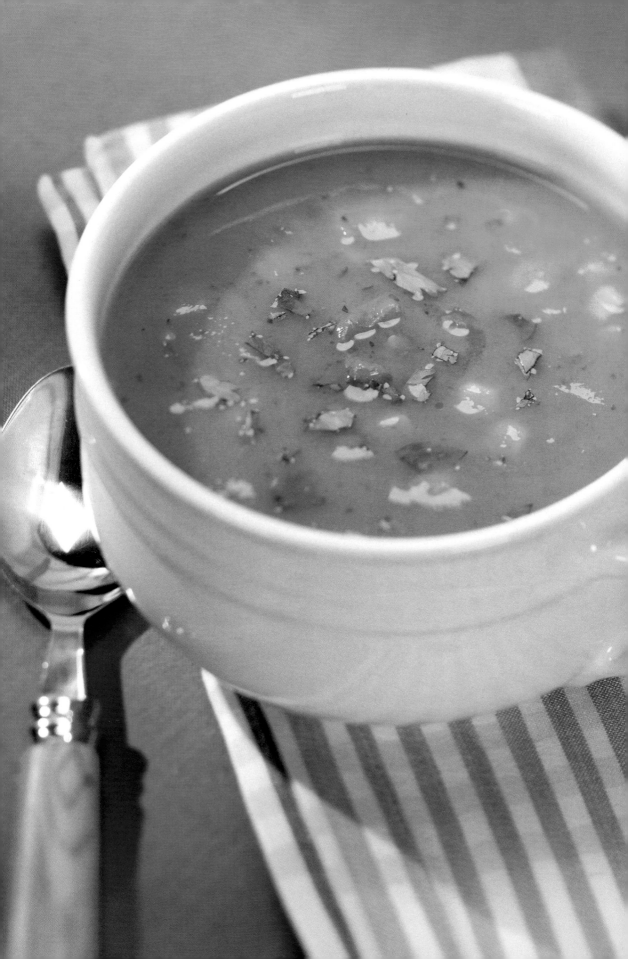

Hearty Beef Soup with Lentils and Barley

Tips

Stewing beef is often used in a soup like this. But I find that it takes a lot of cooking time before it becomes tender — and I'm always in a hurry. So I use more tender cuts of beef: either round or loin. Remember, too, that the smaller the cubes, the faster the meat tenderizes.

This hearty soup is an excellent source of vitamin A and folic acid.

6 oz	boneless round steak, cut into ½-inch (1 cm) cubes	175 g
2 tbsp	all-purpose flour	25 mL
½ cup	chopped onions	125 mL
1 tsp	minced garlic	5 mL
½ cup	chopped carrots	125 mL
½ cup	chopped green bell peppers	125 mL
½ cup	green lentils	125 mL
1	can (19 oz/540 mL) tomatoes, with juice	1
4½ cups	beef stock or chicken stock	1.125 L
⅓ cup	pearl barley	75 mL
2 tsp	packed brown sugar	10 mL
1½ tsp	dried basil	7 mL
2	bay leaves	2
¼ tsp	freshly ground black pepper	1 mL

1. In a bowl coat beef with flour; shake off excess. In a nonstick saucepan sprayed with vegetable spray, cook beef over medium-high heat for 5 minutes or until browned on all sides. Remove meat to a plate; respray pan. Add onions and garlic; cook for 2 minutes. Add carrots and green peppers; cook, stirring occasionally, for 4 minutes or until vegetables are softened.

2. Add browned beef, lentils, tomatoes, stock, barley, brown sugar, basil, bay leaves and pepper; bring to a boil, breaking up tomatoes with back of a spoon. Reduce heat to medium-low; cook, covered, for 45 minutes or until lentils and barley are tender. Ladle soup into bowls. Serve.

FOOD CHOICE VALUES PER SERVING

1½ ■ Starch Choices

2 ◖ Fruit & Vegetable Choices

3 ◖ Protein Choices

NUTRIENT ANALYSIS PER SERVING			
Calories	317	Fat, total	3 g
Carbohydrates	49 g	Fat, saturated	1 g
Fiber	7 g	Sodium	387 mg
Protein	26 g	Cholesterol	31 mg

Santa Fe Sweet Potato Soup (page 40)

Make ahead

This dish can be assembled the night before it is cooked. Follow preparation directions in Steps 1 and 2 and refrigerate overnight. The next day, transfer to slow cooker stoneware and continue cooking as directed in Step 3.

Sophisticated Mushroom Barley Soup

1	cup boiling water	250 mL
1	package (½ oz/14 g) dried wild mushrooms, such as porcini	1
2 tbsp	margarine or butter, divided	25 mL
3	onions, finely chopped	3
6	cloves garlic, minced	6
1 tsp	salt, optional	5 mL
1 tsp	cracked black peppercorns	5 mL
1½ lbs	button mushrooms, sliced	750 g
⅔ cup	pearl barley	150 mL
6 cups	low-sodium beef stock	1.5 L
1 cup	water	250 mL
1	bay leaf	1
¼ cup	low-sodium soya sauce	50 mL
	Finely chopped green onions or parsley (optional)	

1. In a heatproof bowl, combine boiling water and dried mushrooms. Let stand for 30 minutes, then strain through a fine sieve, reserving liquid. Chop mushrooms finely and set aside.

2. In a skillet, over medium heat, melt 1 tbsp (15 mL) butter. Add onions and cook until soft. Add garlic, optional salt and pepper and cook for 1 minute. Transfer mixture to slow cooker stoneware. In same pan, melt remaining butter and cook button mushrooms over medium-high heat until they begin to lose their liquid. Add dried mushrooms, toss to combine and cook for 1 minute. Transfer mixture to slow cooker stoneware. Add barley, reserved mushroom soaking liquid, stock, water, bay leaf and soya sauce.

continued on page 35

FOOD CHOICE VALUES PER SERVING

1 ■ Starch Choice

½ ◆ Fruit & Vegetable Choice

½ ◉ Protein Choice

½ ▲ Fats & Oils Choice

NUTRIENT ANALYSIS PER SERVING			
Calories	138	Fat, total	4 g
Carbohydrates	22 g	Fat, saturated	2 g
Fiber	3 g	Sodium	627 mg
Protein	6 g	Cholesterol	8 mg

3. Cover and cook on Low for 6 to 8 hours or on High for 3 to 4 hours. Discard bay leaf. Ladle into individual bowls and garnish with chopped green onions or parsley, if using.

✤

SERVES 6

Tips

Using a commercially prepared low-sodium chicken stock or vegetable stock reduces the sodium content of this recipe from 1051 mg to 727 mg.

If you have time to make the vegetable stock on page 28, you can reduce the sodium to 127 mg per serving — a saving of 600 mg!

Harvest Vegetable Barley Soup

2 tbsp	margarine or butter	25 mL
1	large onion, chopped	1
3	cloves garlic, finely chopped	3
1½ cups	diced peeled rutabaga	375 mL
½ tsp	dried thyme or marjoram leaves	2 mL
8 cups	low-sodium chicken stock or vegetable stock (see recipe, page 28) (approx.)	2 L
½ cup	pearl barley, rinsed	125 mL
1½ cups	diced peeled sweet potatoes	375 mL
1½ cups	diced zucchini	375 mL
	Salt and freshly ground black pepper	

1. In a large Dutch oven or stockpot, melt butter over medium heat. Add onion, garlic, rutabaga and thyme; cook, stirring often, for 5 minutes or until vegetables are lightly colored.

2. Stir in stock and barley; bring to a boil. Reduce heat, cover and simmer for 20 minutes. Add sweet potatoes and zucchini; simmer, covered, for 15 minutes or until barley is tender. Season with salt and pepper to taste.

FOOD CHOICE VALUES PER SERVING

1½ ■ Starch Choices

½ ◢ Fruit & Vegetable Choice

1 ◕ Protein Choice

½ ▲ Fats & Oils Choice

NUTRIENT ANALYSIS PER SERVING			
Calories	231	Fat, total	6 g
Carbohydrates	34 g	Fat, saturated	3 g
Fiber	5 g	Sodium	727 mg
Protein	11 g	Cholesterol	10 mg

Fassolada (Greek Bean Soup)

2½ cups	dried white kidney beans	625 mL
1 tbsp	baking soda	15 mL
12 cups	water	3 L
1	onion, diced	1
1	large carrot, diced	1
½ cup	chopped fresh celery leaves, packed down (or 2 celery stalks, finely chopped)	125 mL
2 tbsp	tomato paste	25 mL
1 tsp	lemon juice	5 mL
1	medium tomato, blanched, skinned and chopped	1
1 tsp	dried rosemary, basil or oregano	5 mL
1 tsp	salt, optional	5 mL
½ tsp	black pepper	2 mL
¼ cup	chopped fresh parsley, packed down	50 mL
¼ cup	olive oil	50 mL
	Extra virgin olive oil, olive bits, diced red onion, and crumbled feta cheese as accompaniments	

1. In a large bowl cover beans with plenty of warm water. Add baking soda and mix well. (The water will foam and remove some of the gas from the beans.) Let soak for at least 3 hours, preferably overnight, unrefrigerated.

2. Drain beans and transfer to a soup pot. Add plenty of water and bring to a boil. Reduce heat to medium-low and simmer for 30 minutes, occasionally skimming froth that rises to the top.

continued on page 3

FOOD CHOICE VALUES PER SERVING

2 ■ Starch Choices

1½ ◨ Protein Choices

½ ▲ Fats & Oils Choice

NUTRIENT ANALYSIS PER SERVING

Calories	274	Fat, total	8 g
Carbohydrates	40 g	Fat, saturated	1 g
Fiber	10 g	Sodium	481 mg
Protein	14 g	Cholesterol	0 mg

3. Drain beans; rinse and drain again. Scrub pot, cleaning off foam stuck to the sides. Return the beans to the pot; add the 12 cups (3 L) water and place over high heat. Add onion, carrot, celery, tomato paste, lemon juice and tomato. Bring to boil, stirring; reduce heat to medium-low. Cook for $1\frac{1}{2}$ hours at a rolling bubble, stirring very occasionally until the beans and vegetables are very tender.

4. Add rosemary, optional salt, pepper, parsley and olive oil. Cook for another 5 minutes, stirring occasionally, and take off heat. Cover soup and let rest for 5 to 10 minutes. Season to taste with salt and pepper. Serve with any or all of suggested garnishes.

Slow cooker

Cranberry Borscht

6	medium beets, peeled and cut into ½-inch (1-cm) cubes	6
	Leaves from the beets, washed, coarsely chopped and set aside in refrigerator	
4	cloves garlic, chopped	4
1	can (10 oz/284 mL) condensed beef broth (undiluted)	1
4 cups	water	1 L
1 tsp	salt, optional	5 mL
½ tsp	freshly ground black pepper	2 mL
1 cup	cranberries	250 mL
2 tbsp	granulated sugar	25 mL
	Zest and juice of 1 orange	
	Sour cream	
	Chopped dill (optional)	

Tip

For a vegetarian version, substitute concentrated vegetable stock for the beef broth. This soup is also good served hot.

Make ahead

This dish can be assembled the night before it is cooked but without adding the cranberries, sugar, orange juice and zest and beet leaves. Follow preparation directions and refrigerate overnight in a large bowl. The next day, continue cooking as directed in Step 1. Or the soup can be cooked overnight in the slow cooker, finished the next morning and chilled during the day.

1. In slow cooker stoneware, combine beets, garlic, beef stock, water, optional salt and pepper. Cover and cook on Low for 8 to 10 hours or on High for 4 to 5 hours, until vegetables are tender.

2. Add cranberries, sugar, orange zest and juice and beet leaves. Cover and cook on High for 30 minutes or until cranberries are popping from their skins.

3. In a blender or food processor, purée soup in batches. If serving cold, transfer to a large bowl and chill thoroughly, preferably overnight.

4. When ready to serve, spoon into individual bowls, top with sour cream and garnish with dill, if using.

FOOD CHOICE VALUES PER SERVING

1    Fruit & Vegetable Choice

½   ▲ Fats & Oils Choice

NUTRIENT ANALYSIS PER SERVING			
Calories	77	Fat, total	2 g
Carbohydrates	14 g	Fat, saturated	1 g
Fiber	2 g	Sodium	274 mg
Protein	2 g	Cholesterol	5 mg

SERVES 4

Tips

Roasted red peppers taste wonderful, but they require some time to prepare. So when a recipe (like this one) calls for just a small amount, do what I do — use bottled roasted peppers. Look for those packaged in water (not oil) to avoid excess fat. Once opened, a jar of these peppers does not keep for very long, so freeze any unused peppers in small airtight containers.

Roasted peppers make this chowder an excellent source of vitamin A.

Corn Chowder with Wild Rice and Roasted Peppers

1 cup	chopped onions	250 mL
1 1/2 tsp	minced garlic	7 mL
4 cups	vegetable stock (see recipe, page 28) or chicken stock	1 L
1/3 cup	wild rice	75 mL
1 cup	diced peeled potatoes	250 mL
1/8 tsp	salt	0.5 mL
1/8 tsp	freshly ground black pepper	0.5 mL
3/4 cup	low-fat evaporated milk	175 mL
1 tbsp	all-purpose flour	15 mL
1	can (12 oz/341 mL) corn, drained or 2 cups/500 mL frozen corn, thawed	1
1/3 cup	chopped roasted red bell peppers	75 mL
1/3 cup	chopped fresh coriander, basil or dill	75 mL

1. In a nonstick saucepan sprayed with vegetable spray, cook onions and garlic over medium-high heat for 4 minutes or until softened. Add stock and wild rice; bring to a boil. Reduce heat to medium-low; cook, covered, for 15 minutes. Add potatoes, salt and pepper; cook, covered, for 20 minutes or until rice and potatoes are tender.

2. In a bowl whisk together evaporated milk and flour; add to soup. Add corn and roasted red peppers; cook for 3 minutes or until slightly thickened. Serve garnished with coriander.

FOOD CHOICE VALUES PER SERVING

2 ■ Starch Choices

1 ◆ 2% Milk Choice

1 ▰ Fruit & Vegetable Choice

NUTRIENT ANALYSIS PER SERVING			
Calories	233	Fat, total	2 g
Carbohydrates	48 g	Fat, saturated	1 g
Fiber	4 g	Sodium	376 mg
Protein	10 g	Cholesterol	4 mg

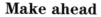

Santa Fe Sweet Potato Soup

2	dried New Mexico chili peppers	2
2 cups	boiling water	500 mL
1 tbsp	vegetable oil	15 mL
2	onions, finely chopped	2
4	cloves garlic, minced	4
1	finely chopped jalapeno pepper, optional	1
1 tsp	salt, optional	5 mL
1 tsp	dried oregano leaves	5 mL
4 cups	peeled, cubed sweet potatoes, about $\frac{1}{2}$ inch (1 cm)	1 L
6 cups	vegetable or chicken broth	1.5 L
2 cups	corn kernels, thawed if frozen	500 mL
1 tsp	grated lime zest	5 mL
2 tbsp	lime juice	25 mL
2	roasted red peppers, cut into thin strips	2
	Finely chopped cilantro	

1. In a heatproof bowl, soak chilies in boiling water for 30 minutes. Drain, discarding soaking liquid and stems. Pat dry, chop finely and set aside.

2. In a skillet, heat oil over medium heat. Add onions and cook, stirring, until softened. Add garlic, jalapeno pepper and salt, if using, oregano and reserved chilies and cook, stirring, for 1 minute. Transfer mixture to slow cooker stoneware. Add sweet potatoes and broth and stir to combine.

continued on page 41

NUTRIENT ANALYSIS PER SERVING			
Calories	175	Fat, total	3 g
Carbohydrates	31 g	Fat, saturated	0 g
Fiber	4 g	Sodium	439 mg
Protein	7 g	Cholesterol	0 mg

3. Cover and cook on Low for 8 to 10 hours or on High for 4 to 6 hours, until sweet potatoes are tender. Strain vegetables, reserving broth. In a blender or food processor, purée vegetables with 1 cup (250 mL) reserved broth until smooth. Return mixture, along with reserved broth, to slow cooker stoneware. Or, using a hand-held blender, purée the soup in stoneware. Add corn, lime zest and juice. Cover and cook on High for 20 minutes, until corn is tender.

4. When ready to serve, ladle soup into individual bowls and garnish with red pepper strips and cilantro.

MAKES 4 SANDWICHES

Tips
To prevent cucumber from turning soggy, assemble sandwiches the same day they are served.

To reduce the sodium content of this recipe, eliminate the salt and, if available, use fresh poached salmon instead of canned.

These nutritious sandwiches are an excellent source of vitamins B_{12}, D, niacin and phosphorus.

Make Ahead
Filling can be prepared through step 1 and refrigerated, covered, for up to two days.

FOOD CHOICE VALUES PER SERVING

2 ■ Starch Choices

2 ◢ Protein Choices

2 ▲ Fats & Oils Choices

Dilled Salmon and Egg Salad on Pumpernickel

3	hard-cooked eggs, finely chopped	3
1	can (7 1/2 oz/213 g) sockeye salmon, drained and flaked	1
1/4 cup	light mayonnaise	50 mL
1	large green onion, finely chopped	1
2 tbsp	chopped fresh dill or parsley	25 mL
1 tsp	grated lemon zest	5 mL
1/4 tsp	salt	1 mL
1/4 tsp	freshly ground black pepper	1 mL
8	slices pumpernickel bread	8
1/2	seedless cucumber, thinly sliced	1/2

1. In a bowl, combine eggs, salmon, mayonnaise, green onion, dill, lemon zest, salt and pepper.

2. Divide salad among pumpernickel slices, spreading evenly. Layer with cucumber slices. Serve open-faced or sandwich together. Cut in half.

NUTRIENT ANALYSIS PER SERVING			
Calories	354	Fat, total	15 g
Carbohydrates	35 g	Fat, saturated	3 g
Fiber	4 g	Sodium	956 mg
Protein	20 g	Cholesterol	175 mg

Tips

Simmer 2 boneless chicken breasts ($\frac{1}{2}$ lb/250 g) in lightly salted water or chicken stock for 10 minutes; remove from heat. Let cool in stock for 15 minutes.

These tasty sandwiches are high in carbohydrate due to the sugar in mango chutney. Reducing the chutney to 1 tbsp (15 mL) can save about 7 g carbohydrate per serving, lowering the ✱ Sugars Choice to $1\frac{1}{2}$.

Curried Chicken Salad Sandwiches

8 tbsp	light mayonnaise	125 mL
2 tbsp	bottled mango chutney	25 mL
1 tsp	mild curry paste or powder	5 mL
$1\frac{1}{2}$ cups	finely diced cooked chicken	375 mL
$\frac{1}{2}$ cup	finely diced unpeeled apple	125 mL
$\frac{1}{3}$ cup	finely diced radishes	75 mL
2 tbsp	finely chopped green onions	25 mL
	Salt	
4	slices thick-cut whole-grain bread	4
	Red leaf or Boston lettuce	

1. In a bowl, blend 6 tablespoons (90 mL) mayonnaise with chutney and curry paste. Stir in chicken, apple, radishes and green onions; season with salt to taste.

2. Spread bread slices with remaining mayonnaise. Spread two bread slices generously with chicken mixture; top with lettuce and remaining bread. Cut in half.

FOOD CHOICE VALUES PER SERVING (1 SANDWICH)

$1\frac{1}{2}$ ■ Starch Choices

1 ◗ Fruit & Vegetable Choice

2 ✱ Sugars Choices

4 ◉ Protein Choices

$1\frac{1}{2}$ ▲ Fats & Oils Choices

NUTRIENT ANALYSIS PER SERVING			
Calories	520	Fat, total	20 g
Carbohydrates	58 g	Fat, saturated	2 g
Fiber	6 g	Sodium	771 mg
Protein	31 g	Cholesterol	72 mg

Pastas, Grains and Wraps

Curried Chicken Coconut Pasta with Apricots and Cranberries

Tips

You can find dried cranberries — as well as dried cherries, blueberries and a whole range of other dried fruits — at bulk food stores, where they are reasonably inexpensive. (But they're not exactly cheap, either.) I buy large quantities and keep them in airtight containers in my freezer until needed. Use them as a delicious alternative to raisins in salads, pastas, rice pilafs and desserts.

Watch portion sizes with dried fruits when you are including them in your meal plan. One-half cup (125 mL) fresh grapes and 2 tbsp (25 mL) raisins contain the same amount of carbohydrate.

12 oz	skinless boneless chicken breast, cut into ½-inch (1 cm) cubes	375 g
2 tbsp	all-purpose flour	25 mL
1 cup	light coconut milk	250 mL
½ cup	chicken stock	125 mL
1 tsp	minced garlic	5 mL
1 tsp	curry powder	5 mL
2 tsp	all-purpose flour	10 mL
12 oz	penne or rotini	375 g
½ cup	chopped red bell peppers	125 mL
½ cup	chopped dried apricots	125 mL
½ cup	dried cranberries or raisins	125 mL
½ cup	chopped green onions	125 mL
⅓ cup	chopped fresh coriander or parsley	75 mL

1. In a bowl coat chicken with 2 tbsp (25 mL) flour; shake off excess. In a large nonstick frying pan sprayed with vegetable spray, cook chicken over medium-high heat for 4 minutes or until cooked through. Remove from pan; set aside.

2. In a bowl combine coconut milk, stock, garlic, curry powder and 2 tsp (10 mL) flour; set aside.

3. In a large pot of boiling water, cook penne for 8 to 10 minutes or until tender but firm; drain. Meanwhile, respray frying pan; return to medium-high heat. Cook red peppers for 2 minutes or until softened. Add apricots, cranberries, coconut milk mixture and chicken; cook for 4 minutes or until thickened and bubbly.

4. In a serving bowl, combine pasta, sauce, green onions and coriander; toss well. Serve immediately.

NUTRIENT ANALYSIS PER SERVING

Calories	432	Fat, total	10 g
Carbohydrates	63 g	Fat, saturated	8 g
Fiber	3 g	Sodium	102 mg
Protein	22 g	Cholesterol	32 mg

Curried Vegetable Chicken Fettuccine

8 oz	skinless boneless chicken breast	250 g
8 oz	fettuccine	250 g
¾ cup	chopped onions	175 mL
¾ cup	chopped green bell peppers	175 mL
½ cup	finely chopped carrots	125 mL
1 tsp	minced garlic	5 mL
1 ½ tbsp	all-purpose flour	20 mL
2 tsp	curry powder	10 mL
1 cup	chicken stock	250 mL
¾ cup	low-fat milk	175 mL
1 ½ tsp	packed brown sugar	7 mL
¼ tsp	freshly ground black pepper	1 mL

1. In a nonstick frying pan sprayed with vegetable spray or on a preheated grill, cook chicken over medium-high heat, turning once, for 12 minutes or until cooked through. Cut into thin slices; set aside.

2. In a large pot of boiling water, cook fettuccine for 8 to 10 minutes or until tender but firm; drain. Meanwhile, in a large nonstick frying pan sprayed with vegetable spray, cook onions, green peppers, carrots and garlic over medium-high heat for 5 minutes or until softened. Add flour and curry powder; cook for 30 seconds. Add stock, milk, brown sugar and pepper; reduce heat to medium. Cook for 2 minutes or until thickened.

3. In a serving bowl, combine pasta, sauce and chicken; toss well. Serve immediately.

FOOD CHOICE VALUES PER SERVING

3 ■ Starch Choices

1 ◆ Fruit & Vegetable Choice

2½ ◉ Protein Choices

NUTRIENT ANALYSIS PER SERVING			
Calories	361	Fat, total	3 g
Carbohydrates	59 g	Fat, saturated	1 g
Fiber	4 g	Sodium	43 mg
Protein	24 g	Cholesterol	39 mg

Pasta Casserole with Mini Meatballs and Tomato Cheese Sauce

Tips

This recipe is a sure-fire hit with kids of all ages. And why not? It combines macaroni and cheese, "beefaroni" and pasta and meatballs — all into one dish! The mini-meatballs are also unusual, appetizing, and just plain fun.

Although many foods contain iron, the type found in grains and vegetables is not as available to the body as the iron found in meat, poultry and fish. In fact, a 3-oz (75 g) serving of lean beef provides as much useable iron as 4 cups (1 L) raw spinach.

MEATBALLS

8 oz	lean ground beef	250 g
1	large egg white	1
3 tbsp	minced onions	45 mL
3 tbsp	plain dry bread crumbs	45 mL
1 tbsp	barbecue sauce	15 mL
1 tsp	minced garlic	5 mL

SAUCE

1/3 cup	mild salsa	75 mL
1/4 cup	tomato pasta sauce	50 mL
1/4 cup	water	50 mL

CHEESE SAUCE

1 cup	low-fat milk	250 mL
1 cup	beef stock or chicken stock	250 mL
2 1/2 tbsp	all-purpose flour	35 mL
1/2 cup	shredded low-fat Cheddar cheese	125 mL
3 tbsp	grated low-fat Parmesan cheese	45 mL
8 oz	small shell pasta	250 g

1. *Meatballs:* In a bowl combine ground beef, egg white, onions, bread crumbs, barbecue sauce and garlic. Form 1 1/2 tsp (7 mL) of mixture into a round meatball. Repeat to make about 36 balls; set aside.

2. *Sauce:* In a nonstick saucepan over medium-high heat, combine salsa, tomato sauce and water. Bring to a boil; add meatballs. Reduce heat to low; cook, covered, for 20 minutes, gently stirring occasionally. Set aside.

continued on page 47

FOOD CHOICE VALUES PER SERVING

3   ■ Starch Choices

1/2   ◆ 2% Milk Choice

1/2   ◗ Fruit & Vegetable Choice

3 1/2   ◑ Protein Choices

1   ▲ Fats & Oils Choice

NUTRIENT ANALYSIS PER SERVING			
Calories	518	Fat, total	17 g
Carbohydrates	58 g	Fat, saturated	8 g
Fiber	3 g	Sodium	469 mg
Protein	32 g	Cholesterol	56 mg

3. *Cheese Sauce:* In a saucepan over medium-high heat, whisk together milk, stock and flour. Bring to a boil, stirring constantly; reduce heat to low. Cook for 4 minutes or until thickened and bubbly. Add Cheddar cheese and 2 tbsp (25 mL) Parmesan cheese; set aside.

4. In a pot of boiling water, cook pasta for 8 to 10 minutes or until tender but firm; drain. In a bowl combine pasta and cheese sauce; pour into casserole dish. Top with meatball mixture; sprinkle with remaining 1 tbsp (15 mL) Parmesan cheese. Bake, covered, for 20 minutes or until heated through.

Leek Pesto over Linguine

1 cup	chopped leeks	250 mL
1 ½ cups	tightly packed fresh basil leaves	375 mL
3 tbsp	grated low-fat Parmesan cheese	45 mL
3 tbsp	toasted pine nuts	45 mL
2 tsp	packed brown sugar	10 mL
1 tsp	minced garlic	5 mL
1 cup	vegetable stock (see recipe, page 28) or chicken stock	250 mL
3 tbsp	olive oil	45 mL
8 oz	linguine	250 g

1. In a nonstick frying pan sprayed with vegetable spray, cook leeks over medium heat for 4 minutes or until softened. In a food processor combine leeks, basil, Parmesan cheese, pine nuts, brown sugar, garlic, stock and olive oil; purée until smooth.

2. Meanwhile, in a large pot of boiling water, cook linguine for 8 to 10 minutes or until tender but firm; drain. In a serving bowl, combine pasta and pesto; toss well. Serve immediately.

NUTRIENT ANALYSIS PER SERVING			
Calories	391	Fat, total	18 g
Carbohydrates	52 g	Fat, saturated	3 g
Fiber	2 g	Sodium	28 mg
Protein	10 g	Cholesterol	0 mg

Sweet and mild or spicy and hot, sausages add a wonderful flavor to meat dishes. Although traditionally made from beef and/or pork, they're now made with other (often leaner) meats, including chicken and turkey. So experiment — and use whatever type of sausage you prefer. Just remember that all sausages have extra fat added, so use them in moderate quantities and be sure to drain the fat after sautéeing.

Rose's Hearty Pasta Sauce with Beef and Sausage

½ cup	chopped onions	125 mL
¼ cup	finely chopped carrots	50 mL
1 tsp	minced garlic	5 mL
6 oz	lean ground beef	175 g
4 oz	Italian sausage, casings removed	125 g
1 ½ lbs	ripe plum tomatoes, chopped	750 g
2 tbsp	tomato paste	25 mL
1	bay leaf	1
1 ½ tsp	dried basil	7 mL
1 tsp	chili powder	5 mL
¼ tsp	salt	1 mL
¼ tsp	freshly ground black pepper	1 mL
1 lb	rigatoni	500 g
¼ cup	grated low-fat Parmesan cheese	50 mL

1. In a nonstick saucepan sprayed with vegetable spray, cook onions, carrots and garlic over medium-high heat for 3 minutes or until onions are softened. Add beef and sausage; cook, stirring to break up meat, for 4 minutes or until no longer pink. Add tomatoes, tomato paste, bay leaf, basil and chili powder. Season to taste with salt and pepper. Reduce heat to medium; cook, covered, for 20 minutes or until thickened.

2. Meanwhile, in a large pot of boiling water, cook rigatoni for 8 to 10 minutes or until tender but firm; drain. In a serving bowl combine pasta and sauce; sprinkle with Parmesan cheese. Serve immediately.

FOOD CHOICE VALUES PER SERVING

2½ ■ Starch Choices

1 ⬕ Fruit & Vegetable Choice

1 ⬤ Protein Choice

1 ▲ Fats & Oils Choice

NUTRIENT ANALYSIS PER SERVING			
Calories	338	Fat, total	9 g
Carbohydrates	49 g	Fat, saturated	3 g
Fiber	3 g	Sodium	202 mg
Protein	15 g	Cholesterol	23 mg

Tip
Look for naturally
brewed soya sauce — it
has a better flavor.

Fusilli with Stir-Fried Beef and Vegetables

1 cup + 2 tbsp	water	275 mL
½ cup	reduced-sodium soya sauce	125 mL
1½ tsp	grated gingerroot	7 mL
1	clove garlic, crushed	1
8 oz	fusilli	250 g
1 tsp	oil, preferably sesame oil	5 mL
8 oz	good quality steak, cut in thin strips	250 g
1 cup	broccoli florets	250 mL
1 cup	finely chopped carrots	250 mL
1 cup	sliced mushrooms, preferably oyster	250 mL
1 cup	thinly sliced onions	250 mL
1 cup	snow peas	250 mL
2 cups	bean sprouts	500 mL
¼ tsp	pepper	1 mL
	Hot pepper flakes to taste	

1. In a saucepan bring water to a boil. Remove from heat; stir in soya sauce, ginger and garlic. Set aside.

2. In a large pot of boiling salted water, cook fusilli 8 to 10 minutes or until al dente. Meanwhile, in a wok or large saucepan, heat oil over high heat. Stir-fry beef until brown. Stir in sauce, broccoli, carrots, mushrooms, onions and snow peas; reduce heat to a simmer and cook for 5 minutes, stirring occasionally. Stir in bean sprouts, pepper, hot pepper flakes and drained pasta; cook for 3 minutes longer. Serve immediately.

This recipe was developed at King Ranch in Toronto.

FOOD CHOICE VALUES PER SERVING

2 ■ Starch Choices

1½ ◨ Fruit & Vegetable Choices

2 ◪ Protein Choices

NUTRIENT ANALYSIS PER SERVING			
Calories	315	Fat, total	4 g
Carbohydrates	51 g	Fat, saturated	1 g
Fiber	4 g	Sodium	789 mg
Protein	21 g	Cholesterol	22 mg

Tip
The good news about pork tenderloin is that it's very low in fat. The bad news is that its low fat content makes it susceptible to drying out when cooked. That's why you should always cook tenderloin quickly over high heat. Use it whole, sliced into medallions and pounded for scallopini, or cut into strips or cubes for stir-fries or kebabs. Keep in mind when shopping that the smaller the tenderloin, the more tender the meat.

Pork Tenderloin with Apricots and Bok Choy over Fettuccine

SAUCE

1 cup	beef stock or chicken stock	250 mL
¼ cup	Asian plum sauce	50 mL
3 tbsp	sweet tomato chili sauce	45 mL
1 ½ tbsp	light soya sauce	20 mL
2 tsp	cornstarch	10 mL
8 oz	pork tenderloin	250 g
1 cup	chopped onions	250 mL
1 ½ tsp	minced garlic	7 mL
1 tsp	minced gingerroot	5 mL
5 cups	sliced bok choy	1.25 L
¾ cup	chopped dried apricots	175 mL
12 oz	fettuccine	375 g

1. *Sauce:* In a bowl combine stock, plum sauce, chili sauce, soya sauce and cornstarch. Set aside.

2. In a nonstick frying pan sprayed with vegetable spray or on a preheated grill, cook pork tenderloin over medium-high heat, turning once, for 15 minutes or until cooked through.

3. Meanwhile, in a large nonstick frying pan sprayed with vegetable spray, cook onions, garlic and ginger over medium-high heat for 5 minutes or until softened. Add bok choy and apricots; cook for 3 minutes or until bok choy wilts. Add sauce; reduce heat to medium-low. Cook for 2 minutes or until thickened; remove from heat.

continued on page 51

FOOD CHOICE VALUES PER SERVING

3 ▣ Starch Choices

1 ◗ Fruit & Vegetable Choice

½ ✳ Sugars Choices

1½ ◑ Protein Choices

NUTRIENT ANALYSIS PER SERVING			
Calories	344	Fat, total	2 g
Carbohydrates	62 g	Fat, saturated	1 g
Fiber	5 g	Sodium	276 mg
Protein	19 g	Cholesterol	23 mg

4. In a large pot of boiling water, cook fettuccine for 8 to 10 minutes or until tender but firm; drain. Slice pork tenderloin thinly crosswise. In a large serving bowl, combine pasta, sauce and pork; toss well. Serve immediately.

SERVES 4

Tip
The sodium in this recipe comes from the cheese, canned tomatoes and salt. By eliminating the added salt you can reduce the sodium content to 800 mg per serving.

Tomato Macaroni and Cheese

2 cups	macaroni (8 oz/250 g)	500 mL
1/2 lb	low-fat Cheddar cheese, preferably old	250 g
1	can (19 oz/540 mL) tomatoes, chopped	1
1 tsp	granulated sugar	5 mL
1 tsp	Worcestershire sauce	5 mL
1 tsp	dry mustard	5 mL
1/2 tsp	salt	2 mL
1/2 tsp	dried thyme	2 mL
1/4 tsp	pepper	1 mL
1/2 cup	dry bread crumbs	125 mL
2 tbsp	margarine or butter, melted	25 mL

1. In large pot of boiling salted water, cook macaroni until al dente, about 8 minutes. Drain well and transfer half to well-greased deep 12-cup (3 L) casserole.

2. Meanwhile, shred half of the cheese and dice remainder. Sprinkle half of each over macaroni in casserole. Top with remaining macaroni, then remaining cheese.

3. Stir together tomatoes, sugar, Worcestershire sauce, mustard, salt, thyme and pepper; pour over macaroni. Toss bread crumbs with butter; sprinkle evenly on top. (Casserole can be prepared to this point, covered and refrigerated for up to 1 day. Bring to room temperature.)

4. Bake, uncovered, in 350°F (190°C) oven for 40 to 50 minutes or until top is golden brown.

FOOD CHOICE VALUES PER SERVING

2½ ■ Starch Choices

2 ◢ Fruit & Vegetable Choices

2½ ◨ Protein Choices

2 ▲ Fats & Oils Choices

NUTRIENT ANALYSIS PER SERVING			
Calories	490	Fat, total	17 g
Carbohydrates	61 g	Fat, saturated	7 g
Fiber	4 g	Sodium	1089 mg
Protein	24 g	Cholesterol	34 mg

Tips
This recipe can be parceled into smaller portions that can be frozen for individual meals — just reheat in the microwave!

Whole wheat pasta is used here, but any type of pasta such as vermicelli or spaghettini can be substituted.

Speedy Singapore Noodles with Pork and Peppers

1 lb	pork tenderloin	500 g
1 tbsp	vegetable oil	15 mL
1	leek, white and light green part only, cut into thin strips	1
2	large cloves garlic, minced	2
1	red bell pepper, cut into thin strips	1
1	yellow bell pepper, cut into thin strips	1
1	green bell pepper, cut into thin strips	1
¾ cup	chicken stock	175 mL
1 tbsp	curry powder	15 mL
¼ cup	bottled oyster sauce	50 mL
2 tsp	cornstarch	10 mL
12 oz	whole-wheat spaghetti	375 g
¼ cup	chopped fresh coriander or parsley	50 mL

1. Cut pork into thin 2- by ¼-inch (5 cm by 5 mm) strips. In a wok or large nonstick skillet, heat oil over high heat. Brown meat on all sides; remove to a plate and set aside. Add leek, garlic, pepper strips, chicken stock and curry powder to skillet; cover and cook for 2 minutes. Stir in oyster sauce.

2. In a small dish, dissolve cornstarch in 1 tbsp (15 mL) water; add to skillet along with pork. Bring sauce to boil; cook, stirring, for 1 to 2 minutes or until pork is heated through.

3. Cook pasta in a large pot of boiling water until tender but firm. Drain well. Return to pot; stir in meat mixture and coriander. Toss to coat well in sauce.

FOOD CHOICE VALUES PER SERVING

2½ ▣ Starch Choices

1 ◪ Fruit & Vegetable Choice

½ ✳ Sugars Choices

3 ◪ Protein Choices

NUTRIENT ANALYSIS PER SERVING			
Calories	389	Fat, total	6 g
Carbohydrates	58 g	Fat, saturated	1 g
Fiber	6 g	Sodium	324 mg
Protein	29 g	Cholesterol	45 mg

Preheat broiler or
set grill to medium-high

Tip

Mango and leeks make
this an excellent source
of vitamins A and C,
niacin and thiamin.

Mango-Leek Sauce over Halibut and Spaghettini

1 cup	chopped leeks	250 mL
1	ripe mango, peeled and chopped	1
1 tsp	minced garlic	5 mL
¾ cup	seafood stock (see fish stock, page 29) or chicken stock	175 mL
3 tbsp	fresh lemon juice	45 mL
2 tbsp	low-fat sour cream	25 mL
1 tsp	Dijon mustard	5 mL
8 oz	halibut	250 g
8 oz	spaghettini or bean noodles	250 g
1 cup	thinly sliced red bell peppers	250 mL
½ cup	chopped green onions	125 mL
⅓ cup	chopped fresh dill (or 1 tsp/5 mL dried)	75 mL

1. In a nonstick saucepan sprayed with vegetable spray, cook leeks over medium-high heat for 3 minutes or until softened. Add mango, garlic and stock; bring mixture to a boil. Reduce heat to medium-low; cook, covered, for 5 minutes or until leeks are tender. Transfer to a food processor. Add lemon juice, sour cream and Dijon mustard; process until smooth.

2. Broil or grill halibut, turning once, for 10 minutes per 1-inch (2.5 cm) thickness or until cooked through. Flake fish with a fork. Meanwhile, in a large pot of boiling water, cook spaghettini for 8 to 10 minutes or until tender but firm; drain.

3. In a large serving bowl, combine spaghettini, fish, red peppers, green onions, dill and dressing; toss to coat well.

FOOD CHOICE VALUES PER SERVING

2½ ▣ Starch Choices

2 ◖ Fruit & Vegetable Choices

2 ◒ Protein Choices

NUTRIENT ANALYSIS PER SERVING			
Calories	351	Fat, total	3 g
Carbohydrates	60 g	Fat, saturated	0 g
Fiber	4 g	Sodium	67 mg
Protein	21 g	Cholesterol	19 mg

Linguine with Salmon, Leeks and Dill

WHITE SAUCE

2 cups	low-fat milk	500 mL
1/4 tsp	nutmeg	1 mL
Pinch	cayenne pepper	Pinch
4 tsp	flour, preferably whole wheat	20 mL
1 tbsp	olive oil	15 mL
1/4 cup	grated Parmesan cheese	50 mL
2	leeks, thinly sliced	2
1/4 cup	white wine	50 mL
2 tbsp	chopped shallots or onions	25 mL
2	cloves garlic, crushed	2
10 oz	linguine, preferably spinach pasta	300 g
12 oz	salmon fillets, skinned, boned and cubed	375 g
3 tbsp	minced fresh dill (or 1 tsp/5 mL dried)	45 mL
Pinch	freshly crushed peppercorns, preferably pink peppercorns	Pinch

1. *White Sauce:* In a saucepan bring milk, nutmeg and cayenne to a boil; remove from heat. In another saucepan, combine flour and olive oil over medium heat; cook, stirring, until blended. Gradually add hot milk mixture, whisking constantly; cook, whisking, until thickened, about 5 minutes. Stir in Parmesan; set aside.

2. In a saucepan combine leeks, wine, shallots and garlic; bring to a boil, reduce heat and cook until vegetables soft, about 10 minutes. Meanwhile, cook the pasta.

continued on page 55

FOOD CHOICE VALUES PER SERVING

2 ■ Starch Choices

1 ◗ Fruit & Vegetable Choice

1/2 ◆ 2% Milk Choice

2 1/2 ◗ Protein Choices

1/2 ▲ Fats & Oils Choice

NUTRIENT ANALYSIS PER SERVING			
Calories	378	Fat, total	10 g
Carbohydrates	48 g	Fat, saturated	3 g
Fiber	5 g	Sodium	161 mg
Protein	23 g	Cholesterol	41 mg

3. In a large pot of boiling salted water, cook linguine 8 to 10 minutes or until al dente. Stir white sauce and salmon into leek mixture; cook just until salmon is barely done, about 3 minutes. Toss drained pasta with sauce, dill and pepper. Serve immediately.

This recipe comes from Cal-A-Vie Spa in California.

Artichoke Cheese Dill Sauce over Rotini

12 oz	rotini	375 g
1	can (14 oz/398 mL) artichoke hearts, drained	1
2/3 cup	vegetable stock (see recipe, page 28) or chicken stock	150 mL
1/2 cup	chopped red onions	125 mL
1/2 cup	shredded low-fat mozzarella cheese	125 mL
1/3 cup	shredded low-fat Swiss cheese	75 mL
1/3 cup	chopped fresh dill (or 1 tsp/5 mL dried)	75 mL
1/3 cup	low-fat sour cream	75 mL
2 tbsp	light mayonnaise	25 mL
2 tbsp	fresh lemon juice	25 mL
1 tsp	minced garlic	5 mL
	Fresh chopped parsley	

Tips

When buying artichoke hearts for this recipe, be sure that they're packed in water, not oil. The oil-packed variety have double the calories and triple the fat — a huge difference!

This recipe is an excellent source of thiamin, niacin, calcium and magnesium.

1. In a large pot of boiling water, cook rotini for 8 to 10 minutes or until tender but firm; drain.

2. Meanwhile, in a food processor combine artichokes, stock, red onions, mozzarella cheese, Swiss cheese, dill, sour cream, mayonnaise, lemon juice and garlic; process until smooth. Transfer to a nonstick saucepan; cook over medium heat, stirring frequently, for 4 minutes or until heated through.

3. In a serving bowl, combine pasta and sauce; toss well. Garnish with fresh chopped parsley. Serve immediately.

FOOD CHOICE VALUES PER SERVING

2½ ■ Starch Choice

1½ ◨ Fruit & Vegetable Choices

2 ◉ Protein Choices

½ ▲ Fats & Oils Choice

NUTRIENT ANALYSIS PER SERVING			
Calories	381	Fat, total	9 g
Carbohydrates	55 g	Fat, saturated	4 g
Fiber	5 g	Sodium	434 mg
Protein	20 g	Cholesterol	19 mg

SERVES 6

Preheat oven to 425°F (220°C)

Baking sheet lined with foil

9-inch (2.5 L) square baking dish, sprayed with vegetable spray

Tip

This lasagna is an excellent source of vitamins A and C, B vitamins as well as calcium, phosphorus, magnesium and zinc.

Roasted Vegetable Lasagna

1	medium sweet potato, peeled and cut crosswise into ½-inch (1 cm) slices	1
1	medium red bell pepper, quartered	1
1	medium yellow or green bell pepper, quartered	1
1	medium red onion, cut into wedges	1
1	medium zucchini, cut into half lengthwise	1
1 tbsp	olive oil	15 mL
1	medium head garlic, top ½ inch (1 cm) cut off, wrapped loosely in foil	1
9	lasagna noodles	9
1 ½ cups	5% ricotta cheese	375 mL
¾ cup	shredded low-fat mozzarella cheese	175 mL
⅓ cup	low-fat milk	75 mL
⅓ cup	prepared pesto	75 mL
¼ cup	grated low-fat Parmesan cheese	50 mL
1 ½ cups	tomato pasta sauce	375 mL
¼ cup	low-fat milk	50 mL

1. In a bowl combine sweet potato, red pepper, yellow pepper, red onion, zucchini and olive oil; toss well. Spread mixture over prepared baking sheet; add garlic. Bake in preheated oven for 45 minutes or until vegetables are tender; remove from oven. Squeeze garlic from skins; mash. Chop roasted vegetables; mix well with accumulated juices and mashed garlic. Set aside. Reduce oven temperature to 350°F (180°C).

continued on page 57

FOOD CHOICE VALUES PER SERVING

- 2½ ■ Starch Choices
- 1½ ◆ Fruit & Vegetable Choices
- 1 ◆ 2% Milk Choice
- 2 ● Protein Choices
- 2½ ▲ Fats & Oils Choices

NUTRIENT ANALYSIS PER SERVING

Calories	528	Fat, total	21 g
Carbohydrates	60 g	Fat, saturated	8 g
Fiber	4 g	Sodium	569 mg
Protein	26 g	Cholesterol	39 mg

2. Meanwhile, in a large pot of boiling water, cook lasagna noodles for 12 to 14 minutes or until tender; drain. Rinse under cold running water; drain. Set aside.

3. In a bowl combine ricotta cheese, mozzarella cheese, ⅓ cup (75 mL) milk, pesto and half the Parmesan cheese; set aside. In another bowl combine tomato sauce and milk; set aside.

4. Spread half the tomato sauce over bottom of prepared baking pan. Top with three lasagna noodles; trim to fit pan (discard trimmings). Add half the vegetable mixture, then half the cheese mixture; spread evenly. Top with three more lasagna noodles; repeat layers. Top with remaining tomato sauce; sprinkle with remaining Parmesan cheese. Bake, uncovered, in preheated oven for 30 minutes or until heated through. Serve.

Singapore Noodles

6 oz	rice vermicelli	175 g
3 tbsp	reduced-sodium soya sauce	45 mL
2 tsp	mild curry paste or powder	10 mL
2 tbsp	vegetable oil, divided	25 mL
1	red or green bell pepper, cut into thin strips	1
5	green onions, sliced	5
2	large cloves garlic, minced	2
3 cups	bean sprouts, rinsed and dried	375 mL
12 oz	cooked, peeled baby shrimp	375 g

1. In a large pot of lightly salted boiling water, cook noodles for 3 minutes. Drain; chill under cold water and drain well. Cut noodles using scissors into 3-inch (8 cm) lengths; set aside.

2. In a small bowl, combine soya sauce and curry paste; set aside.

3. Heat a wok or large nonstick skillet over high heat until very hot; add 1 tbsp (15 mL) oil, tilting wok to coat sides. Stir-fry pepper strips, green onions and garlic for 1 minute. Add bean sprouts and shrimp; stir-fry for 1 to 2 minutes or until vegetables are tender-crisp. Transfer to a bowl.

4. Add remaining oil to wok; when very hot, add noodles and soya sauce mixture. Stir-fry for 1 minute or until heated through. Return vegetable-shrimp mixture to wok and stir-fry for 1 minute more. Serve immediately.

NUTRIENT ANALYSIS PER SERVING

Calories	347	Fat, total	8 g
Carbohydrates	45 g	Fat, saturated	1 g
Fiber	3 g	Sodium	606 mg
Protein	23 g	Cholesterol	166 mg

Pasta Pizza with Goat Cheese and Caramelized Onions

Tip

What's a pasta pizza?
Simple — a pizza with a
crust of pasta, not bread!
The success of this dish
depends on using the
sweetest onions you can
find. Try varieties such as
Spanish, Bermuda or
Vidalia. They're all
perfect — strong in flavor
but not as pungent as
standard yellow onions,
and sweet enough to be
eaten raw. Remember to
store onions in a dry,
dark and cool place;
avoid using plastic bags.

2	large sweet white onions (such as Spanish, Vidalia or Bermuda), sliced	2
2 tsp	minced garlic	10 mL
2 tbsp	packed brown sugar	25 mL
1 tbsp	balsamic vinegar	15 mL
6 oz	wide rice noodles, broken	175 g
1	large egg	1
1/3 cup	low-fat milk	75 mL
3 tbsp	grated low-fat Parmesan cheese	45 mL
2 oz	goat cheese	50 g

1. In a large nonstick saucepan sprayed with vegetable spray, cook onions and garlic over medium heat for 10 minutes. Add brown sugar and balsamic vinegar; reduce heat to medium-low. Cook, stirring occasionally, for 25 minutes or until golden brown and tender.

2. Meanwhile, in a large pot of boiling water, cook rice noodles for 5 minutes or until tender; drain. Rinse with cold water; drain well. In a bowl combine noodles, egg, milk and Parmesan cheese; stir well. Pour into prepared springform pan. Bake in preheated oven for 20 minutes; remove from oven. Set oven heat to broil.

3. Spread onion mixture over baked noodles; dot with goat cheese. Broil for 8 minutes or until cheese is melted.

FOOD CHOICE VALUES PER SERVING

1½ ▣ Starch Choices

½ ▰ Fruit & Vegetable Choice

½ ✱ Sugars Choice

½ ▲ Fats & Oils Choice

NUTRIENT ANALYSIS PER SERVING			
Calories	180	Fat, total	3 g
Carbohydrates	32 g	Fat, saturated	2 g
Fiber	1 g	Sodium	101 mg
Protein	5 g	Cholesterol	42 mg

Angel Hair Pasta with Shrimp in a Tomato Pesto Sauce

½ cup	white wine	125 mL
1 lb	shrimp, peeled and deveined	500 g

SAUCE

1 tbsp	olive oil	15 mL
1	green pepper, chopped	1
1 cup	chopped onions	250 mL
1 lb	mushrooms, chopped	500 g
½ cup	white wine	125 mL
2 lbs	plum tomatoes, finely chopped	1 kg
4 tsp	dried oregano	20 mL
1 tbsp	dried basil	15 mL
1 tsp	honey	5 mL
1	bay leaf	1
1 tbsp	tomato paste	15 mL

PESTO

2½ cups	packed fresh basil leaves	625 mL
¼ cup	walnuts	50 mL
2 tbsp	grated Parmesan cheese	25 mL
1 tbsp	olive oil	15 mL
3	cloves garlic, crushed	3
10 oz	angel hair pasta or capellini	300 g

1. In a small saucepan, bring wine to a simmer. Add shrimp; cook just until pink. Remove from heat; drain, reserving liquid.

continued on page 61

NUTRIENT ANALYSIS PER SERVING			
Calories	460	Fat, total	12 g
Carbohydrates	56 g	Fat, saturated	2 g
Fiber	6 g	Sodium	261 mg
Protein	29 g	Cholesterol	151 mg

2. *Sauce:* In a large saucepan, heat oil over medium-high heat. Add green peppers and onions; cook for 5 minutes. Stir in mushrooms, wine and shrimp cooking liquid; cook for 2 minutes. Stir in tomatoes, oregano, basil, honey and bay leaf; bring to a boil, reduce heat to medium and cook until thickened, about 20 minutes. Stir in tomato paste; cook for another 10 minutes. Meanwhile, make the pesto.

3. *Pesto:* In food processor, purée basil, walnuts, Parmesan, olive oil and garlic until smooth. Measure out $\frac{1}{4}$ cup (50 mL) of pesto for dish; refrigerate or freeze remainder for later use.

4. In a large pot of boiling salted water, cook angel hair pasta for 6 to 8 minutes or until al dente; drain. Toss with shrimp, tomato sauce and pesto. Serve immediately.

This recipe comes from Cal-A-Vie Spa in California.

Preheat oven to
425°F (220°C)

13- by 9-inch (3 L)
baking dish sprayed with
vegetable spray

Tip

This recipe is an
excellent source
of vitamins A and C,
niacin, calcium,
phosphorus and zinc.

Spicy Beef Polenta Layered Casserole

8 oz	lean ground beef	250 g
¾ cup	diced onions	175 mL
2 tsp	minced garlic	10 mL
¾ cup	diced green bell peppers	175 mL
¾ cup	diced carrots	175 mL
2 tsp	minced jalapeno peppers (optional) or ½ tsp (2 mL) dried chili flakes	10 mL
1	can (19 oz/540 mL) tomatoes, crushed	1
¾ cup	canned or frozen corn kernels	175 mL
⅓ cup	sliced black olives	75 mL
1	bay leaf	1
1 tbsp	chili powder	15 mL
1½ tsp	Italian seasoning	7 mL
6 cups	chicken stock or beef stock	1.5 L
1½ cup	cornmeal	375 mL
1 cup	shredded low-fat mozzarella cheese	250 mL
2 tbsp	grated low-fat Parmesan cheese	25 mL

1. In a nonstick saucepan sprayed with vegetable spray, cook beef over medium-high heat, stirring, for 3 minutes or until no longer pink. Add onions and garlic; cook for 3 minutes or until softened. Add green peppers, carrots and jalapeno peppers; cook for 2 minutes. Add tomatoes, corn, black olives, bay leaf, chili powder and Italian seasoning; bring to a boil. Reduce heat to low; cook, covered, for 20 minutes or until thickened and vegetables are tender.

continued on page 63

**FOOD CHOICE VALUES
PER SERVING**

1½ ■ Starch Choices

½ ◆ Fruit & Vegetable
Choice

2 ◉ Protein Choices

1 ▲ Fats & Oils
Choice

1 ✦✦ Extra Choice

NUTRIENT ANALYSIS PER SERVING			
Calories	306	Fat, total	11 g
Carbohydrates	33 g	Fat, saturated	6 g
Fiber	4 g	Sodium	515 mg
Protein	20 g	Cholesterol	38 mg

2. In a nonstick saucepan over medium-high heat, bring stock to a boil. Reduce heat to low; gradually whisk in cornmeal. Cook, stirring, for 5 minutes. Spread half of meat sauce over bottom of prepared baking dish; top with half of polenta. Repeat layers; sprinkle with mozzarella cheese and Parmesan cheese. Cover pan with foil. Bake in preheated oven for 15 minutes or until heated through; let stand for 5 minutes before serving.

Shrimp Risotto with Artichoke Hearts and Parmesan

3 cups	seafood stock (see fish stock, page 29) or chicken stock	750 mL
½ cup	chopped onions	125 mL
2 tsp	minced garlic	10 mL
1 cup	Arborio rice (risotto rice)	250 mL
1 tsp	dried basil	5 mL
Half	can (14 oz/398 mL) artichoke hearts, drained and chopped	Half
8 oz	raw shrimp, shelled and chopped	250 g
¼ cup	chopped green onions	50 mL
¼ cup	grated low-fat Parmesan cheese	50 mL
¼ tsp	freshly ground black pepper	1 mL

1. In a saucepan over medium-high heat, bring stock to a boil; reduce heat to low. In another nonstick saucepan sprayed with vegetable spray, cook onions and garlic over medium-high heat for 3 minutes or until softened. Add rice and basil; cook for 1 minute.

2. Using a ladle, add ½ cup (125 mL) stock to rice; stir to keep rice from sticking to pan. When liquid is absorbed, add another ½ cup (125 mL) stock. Reduce heat if necessary to maintain a slow, steady simmer. Repeat this process, ladling in hot stock and stirring constantly, for 15 minutes, reducing amount of stock added to ¼ cup (50 mL) near end of cooking time.

3. Add artichokes and shrimp; cook, adding more stock as necessary, for 3 minutes or until shrimp turn pink and rice is tender but firm. Add green onions, Parmesan cheese and pepper. Serve immediately.

FOOD CHOICE VALUES PER SERVING

.2½ ■ Starch Choices

1 ◗ Fruit & Vegetable Choice

2 ◖ Protein Choices

NUTRIENT ANALYSIS PER SERVING

Calories	288	Fat, total	2 g
Carbohydrates	49 g	Fat, saturated	0 g
Fiber	2 g	Sodium	254 mg
Protein	19 g	Cholesterol	91 mg

Dilled Salmon and Egg Salad on Pumpernickel (page 41)
Overleaf: Curried Chicken Coconut Pasta with Apricots and Cranberries (page 44)

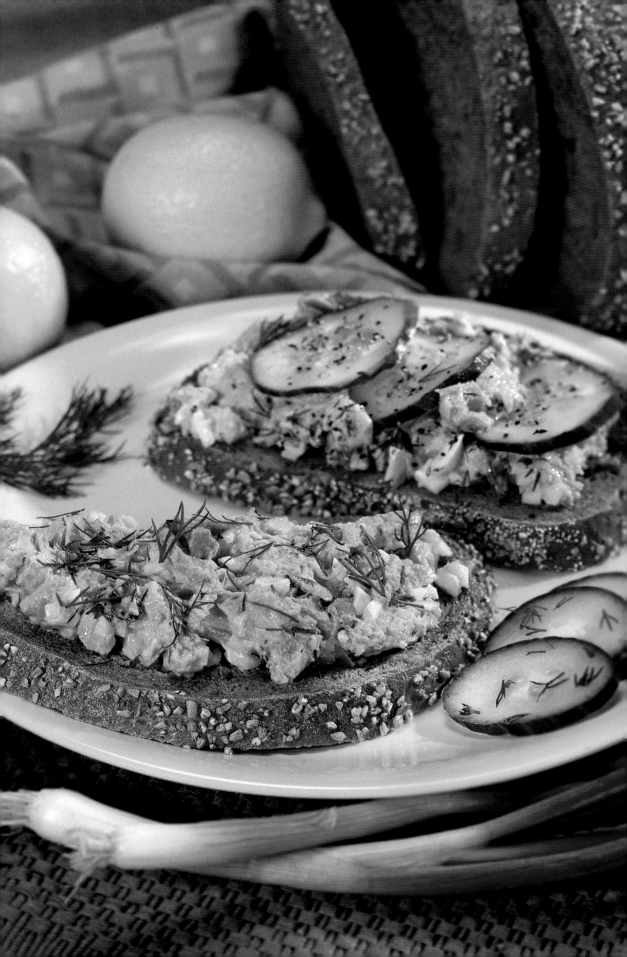

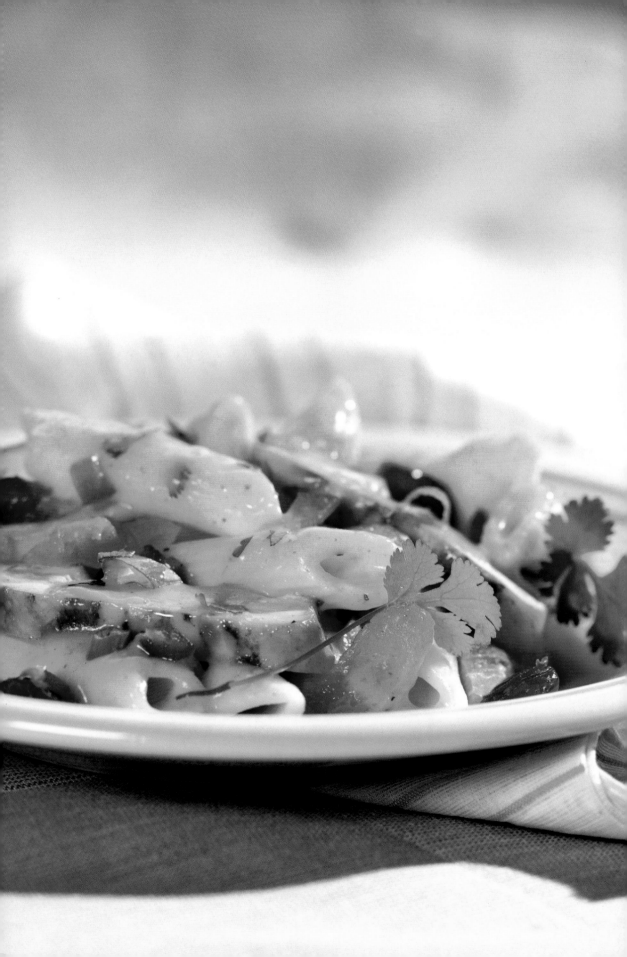

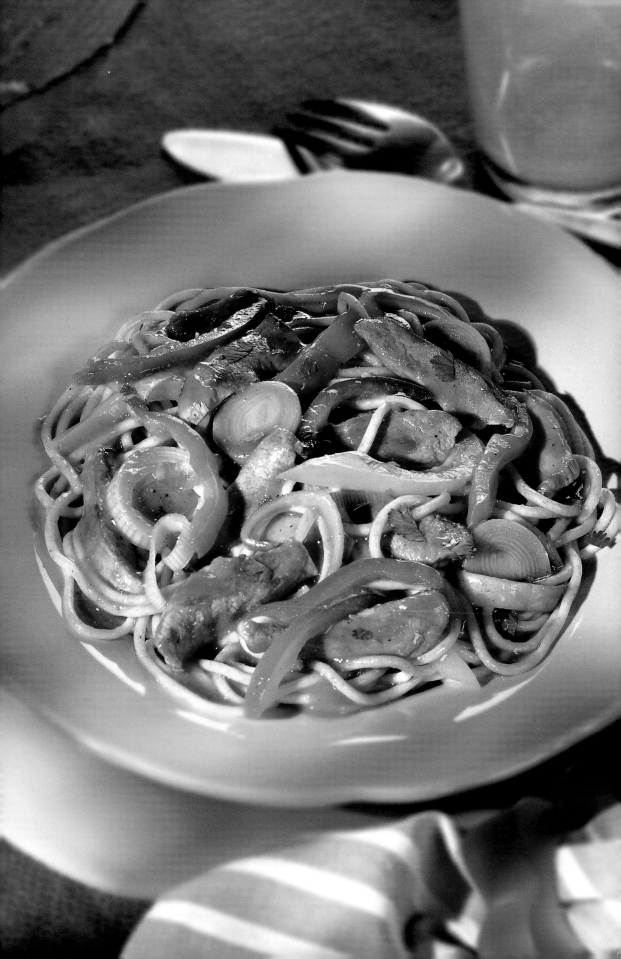

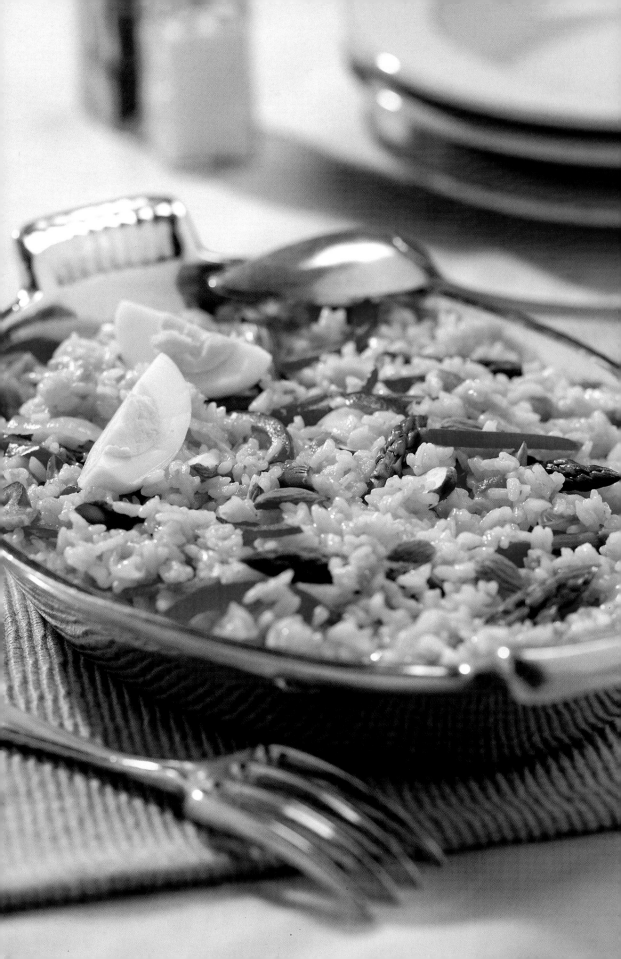

Garden Paella

2 tbsp	olive oil	25 mL
1	sweet red pepper, cut in strips	1
1	onion, finely chopped	1
2	cloves garlic, minced	2
2	tomatoes, peeled and chopped	2
1 1/2 cups	Arborio or other short-grain rice	375 mL
3 cups	chicken or vegetable stock (see recipe, page 28)	750 mL
3/4 tsp	salt, optional	4 mL
1/4 tsp	saffron threads, crushed	1 mL
1 lb	asparagus	500 g
1/2 cup	sliced unblanched almonds	125 mL
2	hard-cooked eggs, cut in wedges	2
	Pepper	

1. In large deep skillet, heat oil over medium-high heat; cook red pepper, onion and garlic for 5 minutes, stirring occasionally. Add tomatoes; cook for about 3 minutes, stirring constantly, until thickened and most of the liquid has evaporated. Remove from heat.

2. Stir in rice to coat. Stir in stock, optional salt and saffron. Return skillet to heat; bring to boil. Reduce heat to low; simmer, covered, for 15 minutes or until rice is almost tender.

3. Cut each asparagus spear into thirds crosswise; arrange over rice. Cook, covered, for 5 to 8 minutes or until rice and asparagus are tender and liquid is absorbed. With fork, stir in almonds. Serve garnished with eggs and sprinkled with pepper to taste.

FOOD CHOICE VALUES PER SERVING

2 ■ Starch Choices

1/2 ◆ Fruit & Vegetable Choice

1/2 ◉ Protein Choice

1 1/2 ▲ Fats & Oils Choices

NUTRIENT ANALYSIS PER SERVING			
Calories	280	Fat, total	10 g
Carbohydrates	38 g	Fat, saturated	2 g
Fiber	2 g	Sodium	297 mg
Protein	10 g	Cholesterol	54 mg

Garden Paella (page 65)
Overleaf: Speedy Singapore Noodles with Pork and Peppers (page 52)

If peanut allergies are a
concern, there are a
number of good
substitutes for the
peanut butter used in the
sauce. Try soya nut
butter, which is made
from dry-roasted soya
beans. It's "soya good,"
you won't know the
difference! Other great-
tasting nut butters
include those made from
almonds, pecans — even
macademias! Try making
your own nut butters by
puréeing roasted dried
nuts with some oil until
the mixture forms a
smooth consistency.

Don't think of these
tortilla bites just as party
appetizers — they make
a great dinner for the
entire family. Don't
bother slicing them; just
"wrap and roll" and enjoy.
Make early in the day,
cover and serve at room
temperature or heat
in the oven at 400°F
(200°C) for 10 minutes.

This is an excellent
source of vitamin C.

**FOOD CHOICE VALUES
PER SERVING**

2	■ Starch Choices
1/2	◢ Fruit & Vegetable Choice
1	◙ Protein Choice
1	▲ Fats & Oils Choice
1	✦✦ Extra Choice

Tortilla Bites Stuffed with Chicken, Pasta and Peanut Sauce

4 oz	boneless skinless chicken breast	125 g
2 oz	wide rice noodles	50 g
1 1/4 cups	julienned red bell peppers	300 mL
1 1/4 cups	julienned snow peas	300 mL
1/2 cup	chopped green onions	125 mL
1/3 cup	chopped fresh coriander	75 mL

PEANUT SAUCE

3 tbsp	peanut butter	45 mL
3 tbsp	water	45 mL
1 1/2 tbsp	rice wine vinegar	20 mL
1 1/2 tbsp	honey	20 mL
1 tbsp	sesame oil	15 mL
1 tbsp	light soya sauce	15 mL
1 1/2 tsp	minced garlic	7 mL
1 1/2 tsp	minced gingerroot	7 mL
3/4 tsp	hot Asian chili sauce (optional)	4 mL
6	8-inch (20 cm) flour tortillas	6

1. In a nonstick frying pan sprayed with vegetable spray
   or on a preheated grill, cook chicken over medium-high
   heat, turning once, for 12 minutes or until cooked
   through; cut into thin slices.

2. In a pot of boiling water, cook noodles for 5 minutes
   or until soft; drain. Rinse under cold running water;
   chop noodles.

continued on page 67

NUTRIENT ANALYSIS PER SERVING			
Calories	287	Fat, total	9 g
Carbohydrates	40 g	Fat, saturated	2 g
Fiber	3 g	Sodium	259 mg
Protein	11 g	Cholesterol	11 mg

3. In a nonstick frying pan sprayed with vegetable spray, cook red peppers and snow peas over medium-high heat for 3 minutes or until tender-crisp. Remove from heat; add chicken, noodles, green onions and coriander.

4. *Peanut Sauce:* In a bowl combine peanut butter, water, vinegar, honey, sesame oil, soya sauce, garlic, ginger and chili sauce; whisk well. Add ¼ cup (50 mL) sauce to vegetable-noodle mixture.

5. Spread about ¾ cup (175 mL) vegetable-noodle mixture evenly over each tortilla; roll up. Cut each tortilla diagonally into 4 pieces. Wrap in plastic and chill or serve warm with remaining peanut sauce for dipping.

Tip
Pork makes this recipe
an excellent source of
thiamin; peppers make it
an excellent source of
vitamin C.

Pork Fajitas with Salsa, Onions and Rice Noodles

3 oz	wide rice noodles	75 g
8 oz	pork or beef tenderloin	250 g
2 tsp	vegetable oil	10 mL
1 cup	thinly sliced red onions	250 mL
2 tsp	minced garlic	10 mL
1 cup	thinly sliced green bell peppers	250 mL
1 cup	thinly sliced red bell peppers	250 mL
1	large green onion, sliced	1
3/4 cup	medium salsa	175 mL
1/3 cup	chopped fresh coriander	75 mL
8	8-inch (20 cm) flour tortillas	8
3/4 cup	shredded low-fat Cheddar cheese	175 mL
1/3 cup	low-fat sour cream	75 mL

1. In a pot of boiling water, cook rice noodles for 5 minutes or until tender; drain. Rinse under cold running water; drain. Set aside.

2. In a nonstick frying pan sprayed with vegetable spray or on a preheated grill, cook pork tenderloin over medium-high heat, turning once, for 15 minutes or until just cooked through. Slice thinly.

3. In a nonstick frying pan sprayed with vegetable spray, heat oil over medium-high heat; add red onions and garlic. Cook for 2 minutes or until softened. Add green peppers and red peppers; cook, stirring frequently, for 2 minutes or until tender-crisp. Add green onion, rice noodles and pork; remove from heat. Add salsa and coriander; combine well.

4. Sprinkle tortillas with Cheddar cheese. Place about 1/2 cup (125 mL) filling in center of each tortilla. Add sour cream; fold bottom end up over filling. Tuck sides in; roll up tightly. Serve immediately.

NUTRIENT ANALYSIS PER SERVING			
Calories	306	Fat, total	9 g
Carbohydrates	37 g	Fat, saturated	3 g
Fiber	3 g	Sodium	376 mg
Protein	18 g	Cholesterol	30 mg

Preheat oven to
425°F (220°C)

Baking sheet sprayed
with vegetable spray

Tips
Seafood or any firm
white fish can substitute
for the salmon.

Substitute chopped
broccoli for snow peas.

Handle cooked
salmon gently, since
it flakes easily.

Make Ahead
Prepare sauce up to
one day in advance.
Keep refrigerated.

Salmon Fajitas in Hoisin Sauce

SAUCE

2 tbsp	hoisin sauce	25 mL
1 tbsp	honey	15 mL
2 tsp	low-sodium soya sauce	10 mL
2 tsp	lemon juice	10 mL
2 tsp	sesame oil	10 mL
1 1/2 tsp	minced garlic	7 mL
1 tsp	minced ginger root	5 mL
1/2 tsp	cornstarch	2 mL
8 oz	salmon, thinly sliced	250 g
1 tsp	vegetable oil	5 mL
1 1/4 cups	halved snow peas	300 mL
1 1/4 cups	thinly sliced red or green peppers	300 mL
1/3 cup	chopped green onions (about 3 medium)	75 mL
3 tbsp	chopped fresh coriander or parsley	45 mL
6	small tortillas	6

1. *Sauce:* In small bowl whisk together hoisin sauce, honey, soya sauce, lemon juice, sesame oil, garlic, ginger and cornstarch; set aside.

2. In nonstick skillet sprayed with vegetable spray, cook salmon over high heat for 2 minutes, or until just barely done at center; set aside.

3. Heat oil in nonstick skillet over medium heat. Add snow peas and red peppers; cook for 4 minutes or until tender. Stir sauce again and add to vegetables, along with green onions and coriander. Cook for 1 minute, or until slightly thickened. Remove from heat and gently stir in salmon.

4. Divide salmon filling among tortillas; roll up and put on prepared baking sheet. Bake for 5 minutes or until heated through.

FOOD CHOICE VALUES PER SERVING

2 1/2 ■ Starch Choices

1 ◗ Fruit & Vegetable Choice

1 ✳ Sugars Choice

2 1/2 ◷ Protein Choices

1 1/2 ▲ Fats & Oils Choices

NUTRIENT ANALYSIS PER SERVING			
Calories	481	Fat, total	15 g
Carbohydrates	62 g	Fat, saturated	2 g
Fiber	5 g	Sodium	613 mg
Protein	25 g	Cholesterol	42 mg

Tips

Quinoa (pronounced KEEN-wah) may be unfamiliar to many North Americans, but it's not exactly new. In fact, it was a staple of the ancient Incas, who described it as the "mother grain." And it seems that they were right! Quinoa contains more protein than any other grain. I like to use it in soups, as part of a main or side dish, in salads and as a substitute for rice.

While it's incredibly nutritious, quinoa can have a slightly bitter taste. But you can eliminate the bitterness by rinsing the quinoa thoroughly, drying it and then toasting it lightly in a nonstick skillet.

A sugar substitute can replace the honey and reduce the carbohydrate by 5 g per serving or eliminate the ½ ✱ Sugars Choice.

FOOD CHOICE VALUES PER SERVING

2 ■ Starch Choices

½ ◆ Fruit & Vegetable Choice

½ ✱ Sugars Choice

1 ▲ Fats & Oils Choice

Quinoa Wraps with Hoisin Vegetables

1 cup	quinoa, rinsed	250 mL
2 cups	vegetable stock (see recipe, page 28) or chicken stock	500 mL
1 tsp	minced garlic	5 mL
1 tsp	minced gingerroot	5 mL
½ cup	diced red bell peppers	125 mL
½ cup	diced snow peas	125 mL
½ cup	diced water chestnuts	125 mL
¼ cup	chopped green onions	50 mL
¼ cup	hoisin sauce	50 mL
¼ cup	light mayonnaise	50 mL
2 tbsp	honey	25 mL
¼ cup	chopped fresh coriander or parsley	50 mL
8	6-inch (15 cm) flour tortillas	8

1. In a small nonstick skillet, toast quinoa over medium-high heat for 2 minutes.

2. In a saucepan over medium-high heat, bring stock to a boil. Add quinoa; reduce heat to medium-low. Cook, covered, for 15 minutes or until grain is tender and liquid is absorbed. Set aside.

3. In a nonstick frying pan sprayed with vegetable spray, cook garlic, ginger, red peppers, snow peas and water chestnuts over medium-high heat for 3 minutes or until softened. Add green onions; cook for 1 minute. Remove from heat; add to quinoa.

4. In a bowl combine hoisin sauce, mayonnaise, honey and coriander; spread over tortillas. Place about ⅓ cup (75 mL) quinoa mixture in center of each tortilla. Fold right side over filling; roll up from the bottom. Serve.

NUTRIENT ANALYSIS PER SERVING

Calories	241	Fat, total	5 g
Carbohydrates	43 g	Fat, saturated	1 g
Fiber	3 g	Sodium	307 mg
Protein	6 g	Cholesterol	0 mg

Casseroles and Other Family Favorites

Tips
Tender beef or veal
can replace the chicken.

Serve over a bed of rice
and with a low-fat
◆ Milk Choice to make
this a complete meal.

An excellent source
of vitamin C, Niacin
and vitamin B_6.

Chicken, Red Pepper and Snow Pea Stir-Fry

SAUCE

½ cup	chicken stock	125 mL
1 tbsp	soya sauce	15 mL
1 tbsp	hoisin sauce	15 mL
2 tsp	cornstarch	10 mL
1 tsp	minced gingerroot	5 mL
8 oz	boneless skinless chicken breasts, cubed	250 g
	All-purpose flour for dusting	
1 tbsp	vegetable oil	15 mL
1 tsp	sesame oil	5 mL
1 tsp	crushed garlic	5 mL
1 cup	thinly sliced sweet red pepper	250 mL
1 cup	sliced water chestnuts	250 mL
1 cup	snow peas, cut in half	250 mL
¼ cup	cashews, coarsely chopped	50 mL
1	large green onion, chopped	1

1. *Sauce:* In small bowl, mix together stock, soya sauce, hoisin sauce, cornstarch and ginger; set aside.

2. Dust chicken cubes with flour. In nonstick skillet, heat vegetable and sesame oils; sauté garlic, chicken, red pepper, water chestnuts and snow peas over high heat just until vegetables are tender-crisp, approximately 2 minutes.

3. Add sauce to skillet; cook for 2 minutes or just until chicken is no longer pink inside and sauce has thickened. Garnish with cashews and green onions.

FOOD CHOICE VALUES PER SERVING

2 ◆ Fruit & Vegetable Choices

2 ◉ Protein Choices

½ ▲ Fats & Oils Choice

NUTRIENT ANALYSIS PER SERVING			
Calories	240	Fat, total	10 g
Carbohydrates	21 g	Fat, saturated	2 g
Fiber	2 g	Sodium	430 mg
Protein	17 g	Cholesterol	32 mg

White-Hot Chicken Chili

Tip
Using regular chicken
stock and adding the
optional salt boosts
sodium to 700 mg
per serving.

2 tbsp	vegetable oil	25 mL
1	onion, chopped	1
1	stalk celery, chopped	1
1 1/4 lb	boneless skinless chicken breasts, cubed	625 g
2	cloves garlic, minced	2
2	jalapeno peppers, chopped	2
1 tbsp	chili powder	15 mL
1 tsp	ground cumin	5 mL
1 tsp	dried oregano	5 mL
Pinch	salt, optional	Pinch
Pinch	cayenne pepper	Pinch
2 cups	low-sodium chicken stock	500 mL
1	can (19 oz/540 mL) white kidney beans, drained and rinsed	1
1/4 cup	chopped fresh coriander or parsley	50 mL

1. In large saucepan, heat half of the oil over medium heat; cook onion and celery for 5 minutes. Push to one side. Heat remaining oil on other side of pan over high heat; brown chicken on all sides, about 5 minutes.

2. Stir in garlic, jalapeno peppers, chili powder, cumin, oregano, optional salt and cayenne; cook, stirring, for 1 minute. Stir in stock; bring to boil. Cover and reduce heat; simmer for 15 minutes. Uncover and simmer for 10 minutes. Stir in beans; cook for 5 minutes, stirring occasionally.

3. Taste and adjust seasoning if necessary. Serve sprinkled with coriander.

FOOD CHOICE VALUES PER SERVING

1/2 ◼ Starch Choices

1/2 ◗ Fruit & Vegetable Choices

4 ◗ Protein Choices

NUTRIENT ANALYSIS PER SERVING			
Calories	247	Fat, total	7 g
Carbohydrates	17 g	Fat, saturated	1 g
Fiber	6 g	Sodium	574 mg
Protein	28 g	Cholesterol	55 mg

Preheat oven to
400°F (200°C)

9-inch (2 L) springform
pan sprayed with
vegetable spray

Tip
Soluble fiber can help
to control blood glucose
and lower blood
cholesterol levels.
Insoluble fibers in
wheat bran and whole
grains help prevent
bowel disorders.

Chicken Cacciatore Over Crisp Barley Crust

CRUST

3 cups	chicken stock	750 mL
¾ cup	pearl barley	175 mL
3 tbsp	low-fat milk	45 mL
2	large egg whites	2
1 tbsp	grated low-fat Parmesan cheese	15 mL
½ tsp	dried basil	2 mL

TOPPING

1 cup	chopped onions	250 mL
1	clove garlic, minced	1
1 cup	chopped mushrooms	250 mL
1 cup	chopped green bell peppers	250 mL
1	can (19 oz/540 mL) tomatoes, crushed	1
½ cup	chicken stock	125 mL
2 tbsp	tomato paste	25 mL
1	bay leaf	1
2 tsp	packed brown sugar	10 mL
½ tsp	chili powder	2 mL
1 tsp	dried Italian seasoning	5 mL
4 oz	boneless skinless chicken breast, cut into ½-inch (1 cm) cubes	125 g
2 tbsp	grated low-fat Parmesan cheese	25 mL

1. *Crust:* In a nonstick saucepan over high heat, bring
   stock to a boil. Add barley; reduce heat to medium-low.
   Cook, covered, for 45 to 50 minutes or until grain is
   tender and liquid absorbed; cool for 10 minutes. Add
   milk, egg whites, Parmesan cheese and basil. Press
   mixture into bottom of prepared springform pan. Bake
   in preheated oven for 25 minutes or until golden at
   edges and firm on top; remove from oven.

continued on page 75

**FOOD CHOICE VALUES
PER SERVING**

1 ◼ Starch Choice

1 ◢ Fruit & Vegetable
   Choice

1 ◙ Protein Choice

NUTRIENT ANALYSIS PER SERVING			
Calories	190	Fat, total	1 g
Carbohydrates	35 g	Fat, saturated	0 g
Fiber	5 g	Sodium	278 mg
Protein	12 g	Cholesterol	15 mg

2. *Topping:* In a nonstick saucepan sprayed with vegetable spray, cook onions and garlic over medium-high heat for 3 minutes or until softened and lightly browned. Add mushrooms and green peppers; cook for 3 minutes or until softened. Add crushed tomatoes, stock, tomato paste, bay leaf, brown sugar, chili powder and Italian seasoning. Bring to a boil; reduce heat to medium. Cook, uncovered, for 20 minutes, stirring occasionally. Add chicken; cook for 3 minutes or until cooked through. Spread mixture over baked crust. Sprinkle with Parmesan cheese. Bake in preheated oven for 10 minutes.

Preheat barbecue grill or
oven to 350°F (180°C)

Tip

If you have time, let
the chicken marinate
for several hours or
overnight in the
refrigerator to intensify
the flavors. To avoid
bacterial contamination,
baste the chicken only
once halfway through
cooking, then discard any
leftover marinade.

Indian-Style Grilled Chicken Breasts

½ cup	plain low-fat yogurt	125 mL
1 tbsp	tomato paste	15 mL
2	green onions, coarsely chopped	2
2	cloves garlic, quartered	2
1	piece (1-inch/2.5 cm) peeled ginger root, coarsely chopped (or 1 tsp/5 mL ground ginger)	1
½ tsp	ground cumin	2 mL
½ tsp	ground coriander	2 mL
½ tsp	salt	2 mL
¼ tsp	cayenne pepper	1 mL
4	chicken breasts (bone-in)	4
2 tbsp	chopped fresh coriander or parsley	25 mL

1. In a food processor, combine yogurt, tomato paste, green onions, garlic, ginger, cumin, coriander, salt and cayenne pepper; purée until smooth.

2. Arrange chicken in a shallow dish; coat with yogurt mixture. Cover and refrigerate for 1 hour or up to 1 day ahead. Remove from refrigerator 30 minutes before cooking.

3. Place chicken skin-side down on greased grill over medium-high heat; cook for 15 minutes. Brush with marinade; turn and cook for 10 to 15 minutes longer or until golden and juices run clear. (Or place chicken on rack set on baking sheet; roast, basting after 30 minutes with marinade, for 50 to 55 minutes or until juices run clear.) Serve garnished with chopped coriander.

**FOOD CHOICE VALUES
PER SERVING**

½ ◆ 1% Milk Choice

3 ◪ Protein Choices

NUTRIENT ANALYSIS PER SERVING

Calories	133	Fat, total	2 g
Carbohydrates	4 g	Fat, saturated	1 g
Fiber	0 g	Sodium	300 mg
Protein	24 g	Cholesterol	59 mg

Chicken and Bulgur Loaf

SERVES 6

Preheat oven to
375°F (190°C)

8- by 4-inch (20 by
10 cm) loaf pan sprayed
with vegetable spray

Tip

This is a wonderful
alternative to traditional
meatloaf. The peppers
help make this recipe
an excellent source
of vitamin C.

¾ cup	chicken stock or vegetable stock (see recipe, page 28)	175 mL
½ cup	bulgur	125 mL
1 cup	chopped red bell peppers	250 mL
1 cup	chopped onions	250 mL
12 oz	ground chicken	375 g
1	large egg	1
1	large egg white	1
¼ cup	ketchup	50 mL
¼ cup	dry seasoned bread crumbs	50 mL
1 ½ tsp	minced garlic	7 mL
½ tsp	dried basil	2 mL
⅛ tsp	salt	0.5 mL
⅛ tsp	freshly ground black pepper	0.5 mL
¼ cup	barbecue sauce	50 mL

1. In a saucepan over medium-high heat, bring stock to a boil. Add bulgur; remove from heat. Let stand, covered, for 20 minutes or until liquid is absorbed and grain is tender. Set aside to cool.

2. In a nonstick frying pan sprayed with vegetable spray, cook red peppers and onions over medium-high heat for 10 minutes or until golden and tender; set aside to cool.

3. In a bowl combine bulgur, ground chicken, egg, egg white, ketchup, bread crumbs, garlic, basil, salt and pepper. On a piece of waxed paper, pat mixture into an 8-inch (20 cm) square. Spread cooled red peppers and onions over surface. Using waxed paper as an aid, roll up mixture from bottom. Lifting waxed paper, gently drop loaf seam-side down into prepared loaf pan. Spread barbecue sauce over top. Bake in preheated oven, uncovered, for 30 minutes.

**FOOD CHOICE VALUES
PER SERVING**

½ ■ Starch Choice

1 ◗ Fruit & Vegetable
Choice

2 ◉ Protein Choices

½ ▲ Fats & Oils
Choice

NUTRIENT ANALYSIS PER SERVING			
Calories	218	Fat, total	9 g
Carbohydrates	20 g	Fat, saturated	0 g
Fiber	3 g	Sodium	262 mg
Protein	15 g	Cholesterol	37 mg

Tips

Bulgar is made of
wheat kernels that
have been steamed,
dried and crushed.

This recipe is an
excellent source of
vitamin C, magnesium,
niacin and B$_6$.

Chicken Bulgur Niçoise

DRESSING

¼ cup	water	50 mL
3 tbsp	fresh lemon juice	45 mL
2 tbsp	balsamic or red wine vinegar	25 mL
2 tbsp	olive oil	25 mL
4	anchovy fillets, drained and chopped	4
1½ tsp	minced garlic	7 mL

SALAD

1⅓ cups	chicken stock or vegetable stock (see recipe, page 28)	325 mL
1 cup	bulgur	250 mL
2	medium red potatoes, scrubbed and quartered	2
8 oz	boneless skinless chicken breast	250 g
8 oz	green beans, trimmed and halved	250 g
1 cup	ripe cherry tomatoes, cut into halves	250 mL
⅓ cup	diced red onions	75 mL
⅓ cup	sliced black olives	75 mL
	Freshly ground black pepper	

1. *Dressing:* In a food processor or blender, combine water, lemon juice, vinegar, olive oil, anchovies and garlic; purée until smooth. Set aside.

2. *Salad:* In a saucepan over high heat, bring stock to a boil. Add bulgur; remove from heat. Let stand, covered, for 15 minutes or until tender and liquid is absorbed. Set aside to cool.

continued on page 79

**FOOD CHOICE VALUES
PER SERVING**

2½ ■ Starch Choices

½ ◧ Fruit & Vegetable Choice

2½ ◎ Protein Choices

½ ▲ Fats & Oils Choice

NUTRIENT ANALYSIS PER SERVING			
Calories	363	Fat, total	10 g
Carbohydrates	50 g	Fat, saturated	2 g
Fiber	7 g	Sodium	286 mg
Protein	22 g	Cholesterol	38 mg

3. Meanwhile, in a saucepan over high heat, cover potatoes with cold water. Cover saucepan; bring to a boil. Reduce heat to medium; cook for 15 minutes or until tender when pierced with a knife. Drain; let cool. Cut potatoes into cubes.

4. In a nonstick frying pan sprayed with vegetable spray or on a preheated grill, cook chicken over medium-high heat, turning once, for 12 minutes or until cooked through. Cut chicken into chunks.

5. In a pot of boiling water, cook green beans for 2 minutes or until tender-crisp; drain. Rinse under cold running water; drain.

6. In a serving bowl, combine bulgur, potatoes, chicken, green beans, cherry tomatoes, red onions and black olives. Pour dressing over; season to taste with pepper. Toss to coat well. Serve.

Best-Ever Meat Loaf

1 tbsp	vegetable oil	15 mL
1	medium onion, chopped	1
2	cloves garlic, minced	2
1 tsp	dried basil	5 mL
1 tsp	dried marjoram	5 mL
¾ tsp	salt	4 mL
¼ tsp	pepper	1 mL
1	egg	1
¼ cup	chili sauce or ketchup	50 mL
1 tbsp	Worcestershire sauce	15 mL
2 tbsp	chopped fresh parsley	25 mL
1 ½ lbs	lean ground beef	750 g
¾ cup	rolled oats *or*	175 mL
½ cup	dry bread crumbs	125 mL

1. In a large nonstick skillet, heat oil over medium heat. Add onion, garlic, basil, marjoram, salt and pepper; cook, stirring, for 3 minutes or until softened. (Or place in microwave-safe bowl; microwave, covered, at High for 3 minutes.) Let cool slightly.

2. In a large bowl, beat the egg; stir in onion mixture, chili sauce, Worcestershire sauce and parsley. Crumble beef over mixture and sprinkle with rolled oats. Using a wooden spoon or with your hands, gently mix until evenly combined.

3. Pack meat mixture lightly into loaf pan. Bake in preheated oven for 1 hour or until meat thermometer registers 170°F (75°C). Let stand for 5 minutes; drain fat in pan, turn out onto a plate and cut into thick slices.

NUTRIENT ANALYSIS PER SERVING			
Calories	345	Fat, total	21 g
Carbohydrates	13 g	Fat, saturated	7 g
Fiber	2 g	Sodium	498 mg
Protein	25 g	Cholesterol	100 mg

Updated Sloppy Joes

Tips

These Sloppy Joes are almost a complete meal. Add a ◆ Milk Choice to complete the meal.

This recipe is an excellent source of vitamin C, iron, zinc, niacin and B$_{12}$.

To reduce the sodium in this recipe to 466 mg while maintaining the taste, replace the tomato sauce with 7 oz (200 mL) tomato paste and the same amount of water.

1 lb	lean ground beef	500 g
1	small onion, chopped	1
1	clove garlic, minced	1
1	sweet green pepper, diced	1
1	sweet yellow pepper, diced	1
1	can (14 oz/398 mL) tomato sauce	1
1 tbsp	red wine vinegar	15 mL
1 tbsp	fresh lemon juice	15 mL
1 tbsp	Worcestershire sauce	15 mL
1 tbsp	packed brown sugar	15 mL
1 tsp	Dijon mustard	5 mL
1 tsp	paprika	5 mL
1 tsp	Tabasco sauce	5 mL
	Salt and pepper	
4	Kaiser buns, split and toasted	4

1. In medium saucepan or large skillet, cook beef, onion, garlic and sweet peppers over medium-high heat, breaking up meat with spoon, until meat is no longer pink, about 10 minutes. Drain off any fat. Stir in tomato sauce, vinegar, lemon juice, Worcestershire sauce, brown sugar, mustard, paprika, Tabasco sauce, and salt and pepper to taste; bring to boil. Reduce heat and simmer, uncovered and stirring occasionally, until thickened, about 20 minutes. Spoon over buns.

FOOD CHOICE VALUES PER SERVING

2 ▣ Starch Choices

1 ◢ Fruit & Vegetable Choice

½ ✱ Sugars Choice

3½ ◪ Protein Choices

2 ▲ Fats & Oils Choices

NUTRIENT ANALYSIS PER SERVING			
Calories	489	Fat, total	20 g
Carbohydrates	48 g	Fat, saturated	7 g
Fiber	2 g	Sodium	1006 mg
Protein	30 g	Cholesterol	64 mg

Baked Curried Beef and Sweet Potatoes

Mashed sweet potatoes contrast nicely with lightly curried ground beef in this comforting supper dish. If you are freezing it, do not add almonds; sprinkle them over top just before serving.

At 4 ▲ Fats & Oils Choices, this may be more than is contained on your meal plan. Eliminate the almonds from the recipe and you can reduce the fat by about 6 g per serving or 1 ▲ Fats & Oils Choice.

Further reduce the fat by eliminating the 1 tbsp (15 mL) vegetable oil. Sauté the onion and ginger in a non-stick skillet with a little water instead.

Nutrient packed, this recipe is an excellent source of vitamins A, E, niacin and B$_{12}$, as well as iron and zinc.

4	small sweet potatoes	4
1 tbsp	margarine or butter	15 mL
	Salt and pepper	
2 tbsp	chopped fresh parsley	25 mL
1 tbsp	vegetable oil	15 mL
1	onion, chopped	1
1 tbsp	minced fresh ginger	15 mL
1 lb	lean ground beef	500 g
2 tbsp	curry powder	25 mL
1 tsp	ground cumin	5 mL
1 tsp	ground coriander	5 mL
2 cups	beef stock	500 mL
2 tbsp	tomato paste	25 mL
1/3 cup	raisins	75 mL
1/3 cup	slivered almonds	75 mL

1. Pierce sweet potatoes several times with fork. Bake in 400°F (200°C) oven for about 1 hour or until tender. (Or peel and cut in large chunks; boil in water for 20 minutes or microwave on High for 7 to 15 minutes.) Peel and mash with butter, and salt and pepper to taste. Stir in parsley. Transfer to 4-cup (1 L) casserole. (Potatoes can be covered and refrigerated for up to 1 day or frozen for up to 2 months. Thaw in refrigerator and bring to room temperature for 30 minutes before proceeding.)

2. Meanwhile, in large skillet, heat oil over medium heat; cook onion and ginger for 5 minutes. Add beef, breaking up with spoon; cook until no longer pink, about 7 minutes. Drain off fat.

continued on page 83

FOOD CHOICE VALUES PER SERVING

2 ■ Starch Choices

1½ ◢ Fruit & Vegetable Choices

3½ ◪ Protein Choices

4 ▲ Fats & Oils Choices

NUTRIENT ANALYSIS PER SERVING			
Calories	583	Fat, total	31 g
Carbohydrates	50 g	Fat, saturated	8 g
Fiber	7 g	Sodium	507 mg
Protein	29 g	Cholesterol	64 mg

3. Stir in curry powder, cumin and coriander. Add stock and tomato paste; bring to boil. Reduce heat and simmer for 20 to 25 minutes or until most of the liquid has evaporated. Stir in raisins and almonds. Taste and adjust seasoning. Transfer to 4-cup (1 L) casserole. (Beef mixture can be covered and refrigerated for up to 2 days, or frozen for up to 2 months; thaw in refrigerator and bring to room temperature for 30 minutes before proceeding.)

4. Reheat both casseroles, covered, in 350°F (180°C) oven for about 30 minutes or until bubbly. To serve, spoon sweet potatoes onto heated platter; make a well in center and spoon in curried beef.

Preheat oven to
375°F (190°C)

Shallow 12- by 8-inch
(2.5 L) baking dish

Tips

Unless you're using
expensive tomato paste
from a tube, what do you
do with leftover canned
tomato paste? You can
freeze leftover tomato
paste in ice-cube trays,
but I prefer to drop
tablespoonfuls (you'll get
10 from a 5 1/2 oz/156 mL
can) onto a baking sheet
lined with plastic wrap
and freeze. When firm,
transfer to a plastic
storage bag or container
and place in freezer.
What's nice about
this method is that
you need only add the
already-measured
amount to your recipe.

This dish is a good source
of vitamin C and an
excellent source of
zinc, niacin and B$_{12}$.

Shepherd's Pie

1 lb	lean ground beef or ground veal	500 g
8 oz	mushrooms, sliced or chopped	250 g
1	medium onion, finely chopped	1
2	cloves garlic, minced	2
1/2 tsp	dried thyme	2 mL
1/2 tsp	dried marjoram	2 mL
3 tbsp	all-purpose flour	50 mL
1 1/2 cups	beef stock	375 mL
2 tbsp	tomato paste	25 mL
2 tsp	Worcestershire sauce	10 mL
	Salt and pepper	
1	can (12 oz/341 mL) corn niblets, drained	1
2 lbs	potatoes (about 6 medium), peeled and cubed	1 kg
3/4 cup	milk or buttermilk	175 mL
2 tbsp	dry bread crumbs	25 mL
2 tbsp	Parmesan cheese	25 mL
1/4 tsp	paprika	1 mL

1. In a large nonstick skillet, cook beef over medium-high heat, breaking up with back of a spoon, for 5 minutes or until no longer pink.

2. Add mushrooms, onion, garlic, thyme and marjoram; cook, stirring often, for 5 minutes or until softened. Sprinkle with flour; stir in stock, tomato paste and Worcestershire sauce. Bring to a boil; reduce heat and simmer, covered, for 8 minutes. Season with salt, if necessary, and pepper to taste.

3. Spread meat mixture in baking dish; layer with corn.

continued on page 85

FOOD CHOICE VALUES PER SERVING

2 1/2 ■ Starch Choices

1/2 ◗ Fruit & Vegetable Choice

2 1/2 ◓ Protein Choices

1 ▲ Fats & Oils Choice

NUTRIENT ANALYSIS PER SERVING			
Calories	385	Fat, total	13 g
Carbohydrates	46 g	Fat, saturated	5 g
Fiber	4 g	Sodium	496 mg
Protein	23 g	Cholesterol	45 mg

4. Meanwhile, in a large saucepan of boiling salted water, cook potatoes until tender. Drain and mash using a potato masher or electric mixer; beat in milk until smooth. Season with salt and pepper to taste. Place small spoonfuls of potato over corn and spread evenly. (The recipe can be prepared up to this point earlier in the day or the day before, then covered and refrigerated.)

5. In a small bowl, combine bread crumbs, Parmesan and paprika; sprinkle over top of shepherd's pie.

6. Bake in preheated oven for 25 to 30 minutes (40 minutes, if refrigerated) or until filling is bubbly.

SERVES 8

Preheat oven to
350°F (180°C)

13- by 9-inch (3 L)
baking dish

Tips

This shepherd's pie rivals the beef version — creamy, thick and rich tasting. Beans provide the meat-like texture.

For a different twist, try sweet potatoes.

Try other cheeses such as mozzarella or Swiss.

Make Ahead

Prepare up to 1 day in advance. Reheat gently.

Freeze for up to 3 weeks.

Vegetarian Shepherd's Pie with Peppered Potato Topping

2 tsp	vegetable oil	10 mL
2 tsp	minced garlic	10 mL
1 cup	chopped onions	250 mL
¾ cup	finely chopped carrots	175 mL
1½ cups	prepared tomato pasta sauce	375 mL
1 cup	canned red kidney beans, rinsed and drained	250 mL
1 cup	canned chickpeas, rinsed and drained	250 mL
½ cup	vegetable stock (see recipe, page 28) or water	125 mL
1½ tsp	dried basil	7 mL
2	bay leaves	2
4 cups	diced potatoes	1 L
½ cup	2% milk	125 mL
⅓ cup	light sour cream	75 mL
¼ tsp	freshly ground black pepper	1 mL
¾ cup	shredded Cheddar cheese	175 mL
3 tbsp	grated Parmesan cheese	45 mL

1. In a saucepan heat oil over medium-high heat. Add garlic, onions and carrots; cook 4 minutes or until onion is softened. Stir in tomato sauce, kidney beans, chickpeas, stock, basil and bay leaves; reduce heat to medium-low, cover and cook 15 minutes or until vegetables are tender. Remove bay leaves. Transfer sauce to a food processor; pulse on and off just until chunky. Spread over bottom of baking dish.

continued on page 87

FOOD CHOICE VALUES PER SERVING

2 ■ Starch Choices

½ ◨ Fruit & Vegetable Choice

1½ ◪ Protein Choices

1½ ▲ Fats & Oils Choices

1 ✦✦ Extra Choice

NUTRIENT ANALYSIS PER SERVING			
Calories	322	Fat, total	11 g
Carbohydrates	42 g	Fat, saturated	6 g
Fiber	6 g	Sodium	466 mg
Protein	15 g	Cholesterol	27 mg

2. Place potatoes in a saucepan; add cold water to cover. Bring to a boil, reduce heat and simmer 10 to 12 minutes or until tender. Drain; mash with milk, sour cream and pepper. Spoon on top of sauce in baking dish. Sprinkle with cheeses.

3. Bake, uncovered, 20 minutes or until hot.

Make ahead
This dish can be partially prepared the night before it is cooked. Make mashed potatoes, cover and refrigerate. Complete Steps 1 and 2, chilling cooked meat and onion mixture separately. Refrigerate overnight. The next morning, continue cooking as directed in Step 3.

Shepherd's Pie with Creamy Corn Filling

1 tbsp	vegetable oil	15 mL
1 lb	lean ground beef	500 g
2	onions, finely chopped	2
4	cloves garlic, minced	4
2 tsp	paprika	10 mL
1 tsp	salt, optional	5 mL
1/2 tsp	cracked black peppercorns	2 mL
2 tbsp	all-purpose flour	25 mL
1 cup	condensed beef broth (undiluted)	250 mL
2 tbsp	tomato paste	25 mL
1	can (19 oz/540 mL) cream-style corn	1
4 cups	mashed potatoes, seasoned with 1 tbsp (15 mL) butter, 1/2 tsp (2 mL) salt, optional and 1/4 tsp (1 mL) black pepper	1 L
1/4 cup	shredded Cheddar cheese	50 mL

1. In a skillet, heat oil over medium-high heat. Add beef and cook, breaking up with the back of a spoon, until meat is no longer pink. Using a slotted spoon, transfer to slow cooker stoneware. Drain off liquid.

2. Reduce heat to medium. Add onions to pan and cook until softened. Add garlic, paprika, optional salt and pepper and cook, stirring, for 1 minute. Sprinkle flour over mixture, stir and cook for 1 minute. Add beef broth and tomato paste, stir to combine and cook, stirring, until thickened.

3. Transfer mixture to slow cooker stoneware. Spread corn evenly over mixture and top with mashed potatoes. Sprinkle cheese on top, cover and cook on Low for 4 to 6 hours or on High for 3 to 4 hours, until hot and bubbly.

FOOD CHOICE VALUES PER SERVING

2 1/2 ■ Starch Choices

1/2 ◆ Fruit & Vegetable Choice

1/2 ✴ Sugars Choices

2 1/2 ◿ Protein Choices

1 1/2 ▲ Fats & Oils Choices

NUTRIENT ANALYSIS PER SERVING			
Calories	422	Fat, total	16 g
Carbohydrates	51 g	Fat, saturated	7 g
Fiber	4 g	Sodium	601 mg
Protein	23 g	Cholesterol	53 mg

Slow cooker

Make ahead

This dish can be partially prepared the night before it is cooked. Complete Step 2, heating 1 tbsp (15 mL) oil in pan before softening onions, carrots and celery. Cover and refrigerate mixture overnight. The next morning, brown steak (Step 1), or skip this step and place steak directly in stoneware. Continue cooking as directed. Alternatively, cook steak overnight and refrigerate. When ready to serve, bring to a boil in a large skillet and simmer for 10 minutes, until meat is heated through and sauce is hot and bubbling.

Saucy Swiss Steak

1 tbsp	vegetable oil	15 mL
2 lbs	round steak or "simmering" steak	1 kg
2	medium onions, finely chopped	2
1/4 cup	thinly sliced carrots	50 mL
1	small carrot, thinly sliced, about 1/4 cup (50 mL)	1
I	small stalk celery, thinly sliced, about 1/4 cup (50 mL)	1
1/2 tsp	salt	2 mL
1/4 tsp	black pepper	1 mL
2 tbsp	all-purpose flour	25 mL
1	can (28 oz/796 mL) plum tomatoes, drained and chopped, 1/2 cup (125 mL) juice reserved	1
1 tbsp	Worcestershire sauce	15 mL
1	bay leaf	1

1. In a skillet, heat oil over medium-high heat. Add steak, in pieces, if necessary, and brown on both sides. Transfer to slow cooker stoneware.

2. Reduce heat to medium-low. Add onion, carrots, celery, salt and pepper to pan. Cover and cook until vegetables are softened, about 8 minutes. Sprinkle flour over vegetables and cook for 1 minute, stirring. Add tomatoes, reserved juice and Worcestershire sauce. Bring to a boil, stirring until slightly thickened. Add bay leaf.

3. Pour tomato mixture over steak and cook on Low for 8 to 10 hours or on High for 4 to 5 hours, until meat is tender. Discard bay leaf.

FOOD CHOICE VALUES PER SERVING

1 🍃 Fruit & Vegetable Choice

4 🥩 Protein Choices

NUTRIENT ANALYSIS PER SERVING			
Calories	196	Fat, total	4 g
Carbohydrates	11 g	Fat, saturated	1 g
Fiber	2 g	Sodium	330 mg
Protein	28 g	Cholesterol	49 mg

Old-Fashioned Beef Stew

Tips
This comfort food is an excellent source of nutrients including vitamins A and C, B vitamins and iron, phosphorus, magnesium and zinc.

If you add the salt and use regular beef stock, sodium is 854 mg per serving.

¼ cup	all-purpose flour	50 mL
1 tsp	salt, optional	5 mL
½ tsp	pepper	2 mL
2 tbsp	vegetable oil (approx.)	25 mL
1½ lbs	stewing beef, cut into cubes 1½ inches (4 cm) square	750 g
2	medium onions, chopped	2
3	cloves garlic, finely chopped	3
1 tsp	dried thyme	5 mL
1 tsp	dried marjoram	5 mL
1	bay leaf	1
1 cup	red wine or additional beef stock	250 mL
3 tbsp	tomato paste	45 mL
3 cups	low-sodium beef stock (approx.)	750 mL
5	carrots	5
2	stalks celery	2
1½ lbs	potatoes (about 5)	750 g
12 oz	green beans	375 g
¼ cup	chopped fresh parsley	50 mL

1. Combine flour, optional salt and pepper in a heavy plastic bag. In batches, add beef to flour mixture and toss to coat. Transfer to a plate. Reserve remaining flour mixture.

2. In a Dutch oven, heat half the oil over medium-high heat; cook beef in batches, adding more oil as needed, until browned all over. Transfer to a plate.

3. Reduce heat to medium-low. Add onions, garlic, thyme, marjoram, bay leaf and remaining flour to pan; cook, stirring, for 4 minutes or until softened. Add wine and tomato paste; cook, stirring, to scrape up brown bits. Return beef and any accumulated juices to pan; pour in stock.

continued on page 91

NUTRIENT ANALYSIS PER SERVING			
Calories	419	Fat, total	13 g
Carbohydrates	38 g	Fat, saturated	4 g
Fiber	5 g	Sodium	359 mg
Protein	32 g	Cholesterol	55 mg

4. Bring to a boil, stirring, until slightly thickened. Reduce heat, cover and simmer over medium-low heat, stirring occasionally, for 1 hour.

5. Meanwhile, peel carrots and halve lengthwise. Cut carrots and celery into $1\frac{1}{2}$-inch (4 cm) chunks. Peel potatoes and quarter. Add vegetables to pan. Cover and simmer for 30 minutes.

6. Trim ends of beans and cut into 2-inch (5 cm) lengths. Stir into stew mixture, adding more stock if necessary, until vegetables are just covered. Cover and simmer for 30 minutes more or until vegetables are tender. Remove bay leaf and stir in parsley. Adjust seasoning with salt and pepper to taste.

Veal Paprikash

Tips
Fettuccine or other long noodles make a delicious companion to this creamy veal in mushroom sauce.

The most flavorful paprika comes from Hungary where it ranges in strength from mild (sweet) to hot.

This recipe is an excellent source of iron, zinc, phosphorus and B vitamins.

2 tbsp	vegetable oil	25 mL
1 lb	grain-fed veal scallops or boneless beef sirloin, cut into thin strips	500 g
4 cups	quartered mushrooms (about 12 oz/375 g)	1 L
1	large onion, halved lengthwise and thinly sliced	1
2	cloves garlic, minced	2
4 tsp	sweet Hungarian paprika	20 mL
1/2 tsp	dried marjoram	2 mL
1/2 tsp	salt	2 mL
1/4 tsp	pepper	1 mL
1 tbsp	all-purpose flour	15 mL
3/4 cup	chicken stock	175 mL
1/2 cup	sour cream	125 mL
	Salt and pepper	

1. In a large nonstick skillet, heat half the oil over high heat; stir-fry veal in 2 batches, each for 3 minutes or until browned but still pink inside. Transfer to a plate along with pan juices; keep warm.

2. Reduce heat to medium. Add remaining oil. Add mushrooms, onion, garlic, paprika, marjoram, salt and pepper; cook, stirring often, for 7 minutes or until lightly colored.

3. Sprinkle mushroom mixture with flour; pour in stock. Cook, stirring, for 2 minutes or until thickened. Stir in sour cream. Return veal and accumulated juices to pan; cook 1 minute more or until heated through. Adjust seasoning with salt and pepper to taste; serve immediately.

FOOD CHOICE VALUES PER SERVING

1/2   ◖ Fruit & Vegetable Choice

1/2   ◆ 2% Milk Choice

4   ◉ Protein Choices

1   ••• Extra Choice

NUTRIENT ANALYSIS PER SERVING			
Calories	266	Fat, total	11 g
Carbohydrates	12 g	Fat, saturated	1 g
Fiber	2 g	Sodium	462 mg
Protein	30 g	Cholesterol	107 mg

SERVES 4

Tip
Enjoy this quick skillet supper with a green salad and low-fat dressing. Finish with sliced fruit topped with a fat-free, no sugar added yogurt.

Tex-Mex Pork Chops with Black Bean-Corn Salsa

4	pork chops	4
1	clove garlic, minced	1
2 tsp	chili powder	10 mL
1 tsp	ground cumin	5 mL
1 tsp	dried oregano	5 mL
1/4 tsp	hot pepper flakes	1 mL
	Salt and pepper	
1 tbsp	vegetable oil	15 mL
1	can (19 oz/540 mL) black beans, drained and rinsed	1
1 cup	corn kernels (frozen or canned)	250 mL
1 cup	bottled salsa (preferably chunky)	250 mL
1/3 cup	chopped fresh coriander	75 mL

1. Trim any fat from chops. Combine garlic, chili powder, cumin, oregano, hot pepper flakes and 1/4 tsp (1 mL) each of the salt and pepper; rub all over chops.

2. In large heavy skillet, heat oil over medium-high heat; cook chops for 5 minutes on each side; reducing heat if starting to stick. Remove to plate.

3. Remove any fat and burnt bits from pan. Return chops and any juices. Add beans, corn and salsa. (Recipe can be prepared to this point, covered and refrigerated for up to 8 hours. Bring to room temperature for 30 minutes before proceeding.)

4. Bring to boil, reduce heat and simmer for about 8 minutes or until sauce is hot. Taste and adjust seasoning if necessary. Serve sprinkled with coriander.

FOOD CHOICE VALUES PER SERVING

2 ■ Starch Choices

1/2 ◨ Fruit & Vegetable Choice

4 ◨ Protein Choices

NUTRIENT ANALYSIS PER SERVING			
Calories	400	Fat, total	10 g
Carbohydrates	45 g	Fat, saturated	2 g
Fiber	12 g	Sodium	218 mg
Protein	35 g	Cholesterol	51 mg

Preheat oven to
350°F (180°C)

Roasting pan with rack

Tips

It may appear that you
have too much stuffing
when you first tie the
pork. But once all the
strings are in place, it's
easy to enclose the meat
completely around
the fruit mixture.

This delicious roast
is likely to be more
🙂 Protein Choices than
on most meal plans.
Either choose a smaller
serving size or balance
it by taking less protein
at another meal.

Company Pork Roast with Fruit Stuffing

STUFFING

1 tbsp	margarine or butter	15 mL
⅓ cup	chopped green onions	75 mL
1 tsp	ground cumin	5 mL
½ tsp	curry powder	2 mL
1 cup	chopped mixed dried fruits, such as apricots, prunes, apples, cranberries	250 mL
½ cup	soft bread crumbs	125 mL
1 tsp	grated orange rind	5 mL
1	egg, beaten	1
	Salt and pepper	
3 lbs	boneless pork loin roast	1.5 kg
2 tsp	vegetable oil	10 mL
1	large clove garlic, minced	1
1 tsp	rubbed sage	5 mL
½ tsp	dried thyme	2 mL
1 tbsp	all-purpose flour	15 mL
½ cup	white wine or chicken stock	125 mL
¾ cup	chicken stock	175 mL

1. *Stuffing:* In a small skillet, melt butter over medium heat. Add green onions, cumin and curry powder; cook, stirring, for 2 minutes or until softened.

2. In a bowl combine onion mixture, dried fruits, bread crumbs, orange rind and egg; season with salt and pepper.

continued on page 95

FOOD CHOICE VALUES PER SERVING

1   🍎 Fruit & Vegetable Choices

5   🙂 Protein Choices

NUTRIENT ANALYSIS PER SERVING			
Calories	258	Fat, total	8 g
Carbohydrates	12 g	Fat, saturated	3 g
Fiber	1 g	Sodium	173 mg
Protein	32 g	Cholesterol	119 mg

3. Remove strings from pork roast; unfold roast and trim excess fat. Place pork roast, boned side up, on work surface. Cover with plastic wrap and pound using a meat mallet to flatten slightly. Season with salt and pepper; spread stuffing down center of meat. Roll the pork around the stuffing and tie securely at 6 intervals with butcher's string.

4. Place roast on rack in roasting pan. In a small bowl, combine oil, garlic, sage and thyme; spread over pork roast and season with salt and pepper.

5. Roast in preheated oven for $1\frac{1}{2}$ to $1\frac{3}{4}$ hours or until meat thermometer registers 160°F (70°C).

6. Remove roast to cutting board; tent with foil and let stand for 10 minutes before carving.

7. Pour off fat in pan. Place over medium heat; sprinkle with flour. Cook, stirring, for 1 minute or until lightly colored. Add wine or stock; cook until partially reduced. Add stock and bring to a boil, scraping any brown bits from bottom of pan. Season with salt and pepper to taste. Strain sauce through a fine sieve into a warm sauceboat. Cut pork into thick slices and serve accompanied with gravy.

Tips

Here's a soothing dish to serve for casual get-togethers. This stew requires no more preparation time than a stir-fry or one-pot dish. Cutting the meat into smaller pieces also shortens the cooking time.

Sodium content totals 1097 mg per serving with optional salt.

This nutritious recipe is an excellent source of 8 vitamins and 3 minerals.

Variation

Lean stewing beef can be substituted for the pork. For a vegetarian dish, replace meat with cubes of firm tofu. Add along with kidney beans.

Make-Ahead Southwestern Pork Stew

4 tsp	olive oil, divided	20 mL
1 lb	lean stewing pork, cut into ¾-inch (2 cm) cubes	500 g
2	medium onions, chopped	2
3	cloves garlic, finely chopped	3
4 tsp	chili powder	20 mL
1½ tsp	dried oregano leaves	7 mL
1 tsp	ground cumin	5 mL
¾ tsp	salt, optional	4 mL
½ tsp	hot pepper flakes	2 mL
3 tbsp	all-purpose flour	45 mL
2 cups	low-sodium beef or chicken stock	500 mL
1	can (28 oz/796 mL) tomatoes, including juice, chopped	1
2	bell peppers (assorted colors), cubed	2
2 cups	frozen corn kernels	500 mL
1	can (19 oz/540 mL) kidney beans or black beans, drained and rinsed	1
	Chopped cilantro (optional)	

1. In a Dutch oven or large saucepan, heat 2 tsp (10 mL) oil over high heat; brown pork in batches. Transfer to a plate. Add remaining oil to pan; reduce heat to medium. Add onions, garlic, chili powder, oregano, cumin, optional salt and hot pepper flakes; cook, stirring, for 2 minutes or until softened.

2. Sprinkle with flour; stir in stock and tomatoes with juice. Bring to a boil, stirring until thickened. Return pork and accumulated juices to pan; reduce heat, cover and simmer for 1 hour or until meat is tender.

continued on page 97

NUTRIENT ANALYSIS PER SERVING			
Calories	384	Fat, total	9 g
Carbohydrates	51 g	Fat, saturated	2 g
Fiber	10 g	Sodium	737 mg
Protein	30 g	Cholesterol	42 mg

Indian-Style Grilled Chicken Breasts (page 76)
Overleaf: Shepherd's Pie
with Creamy Corn Filling (page 88)

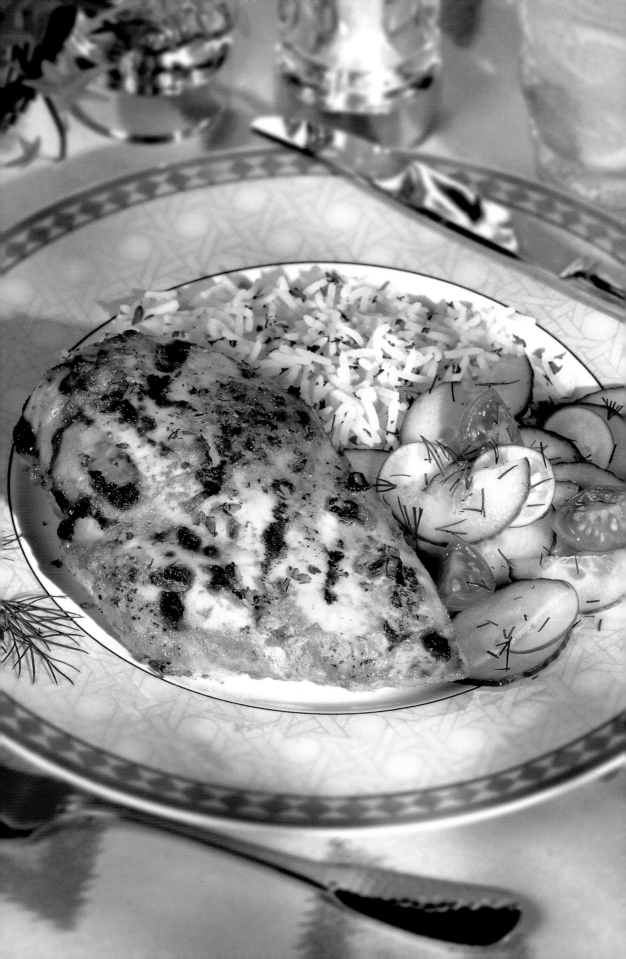

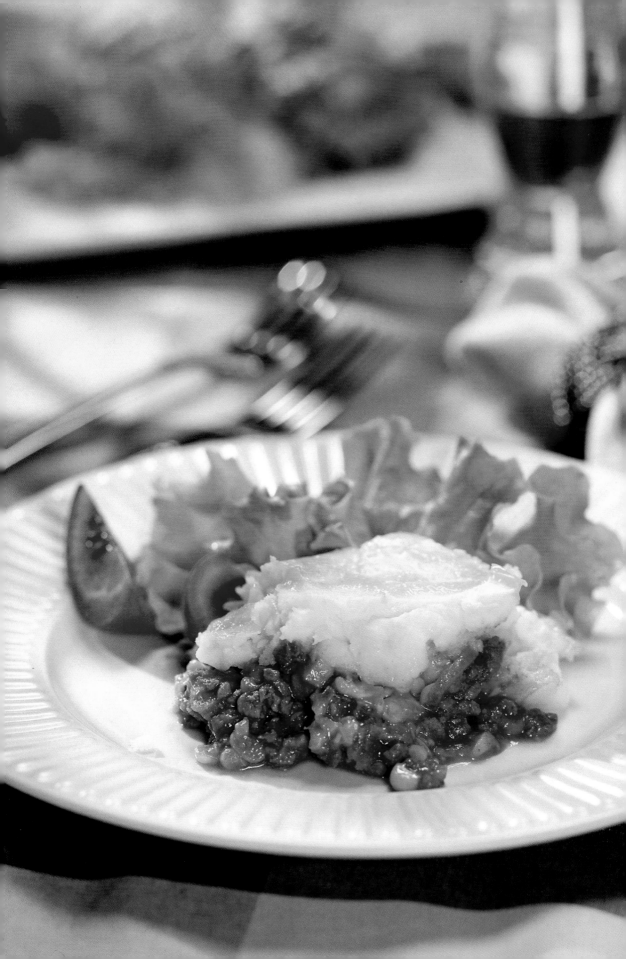

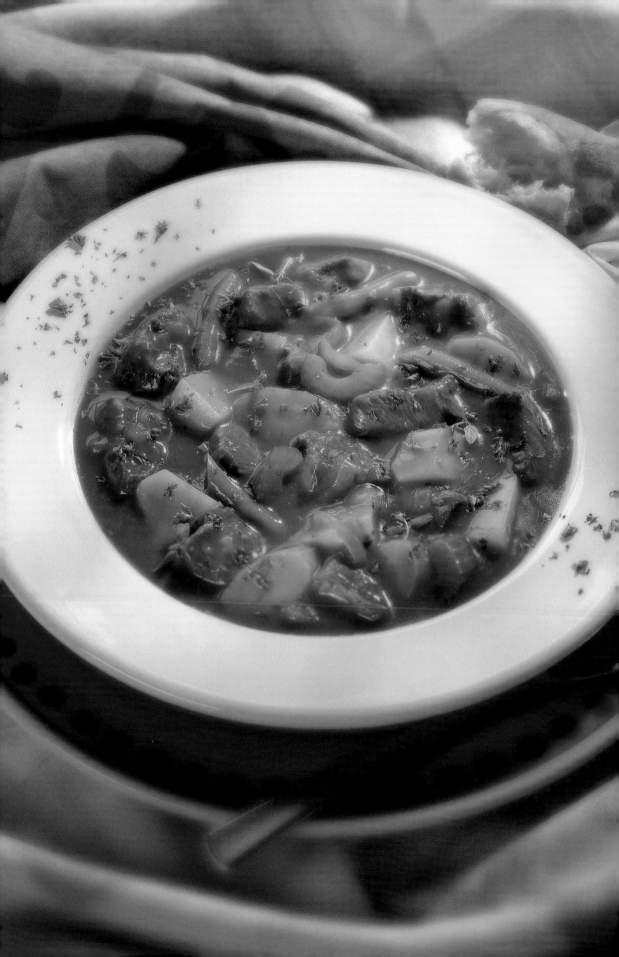

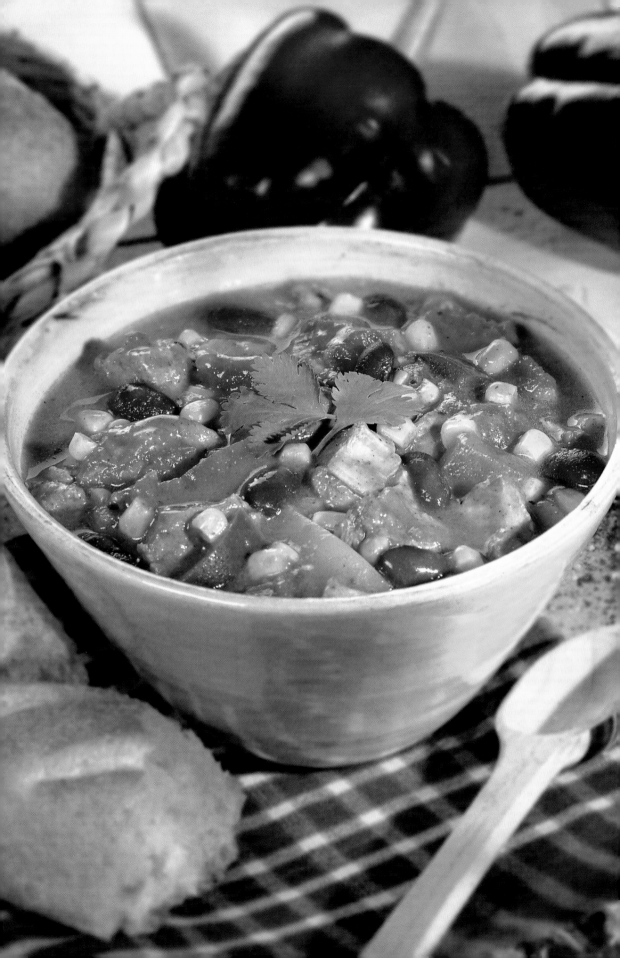

3. Add bell peppers, corn and kidney beans; simmer, covered, for 15 minutes or until vegetables are tender. Garnish with chopped cilantro, if desired.

Pork with Pears, Honey and Thyme

SERVES 4

Tips

Apples have always been paired with pork but pears deserve equal treatment. Here they make an especially delicious companion to this versatile meat.

Serve with rice and a steamed green vegetable such as snow peas, along with red pepper or broccoli.

You can replace the honey with a sugar substitute to save 5 g carbohydrate, or ½ ✳ Sugars Choice.

1 tbsp	vegetable oil	15 mL
1 lb	thin boneless pork loin chops (about 8)	500 g
2	pears, peeled, cored and thinly sliced	2
3	green onions, chopped	3
1 tbsp	honey	15 mL
½ tsp	dried thyme	2 mL
½ cup	chicken stock	125 mL
1 tbsp	cider vinegar	15 mL
1 tsp	cornstarch	5 mL
¼ tsp	salt	1 mL
¼ tsp	pepper	1 mL

1. In a large nonstick skillet, heat oil over medium-high heat; brown pork for 2 minutes on each side. Remove to a plate and keep warm. Add pears, green onions, honey and thyme to skillet; cook, stirring, for 2 to 3 minutes or until pears are softened.

2. Meanwhile, in a bowl, combine stock, vinegar, cornstarch, salt and pepper. Pour into skillet; cook, stirring, until slightly thickened. Return pork and any accumulated juices to skillet and cook, turning occasionally, for 1 to 2 minutes or until heated through.

FOOD CHOICE VALUES PER SERVING

1	■ Starch Choice
½	✳ Sugars Choice
3½	◙ Protein Choices

NUTRIENT ANALYSIS PER SERVING			
Calories	265	Fat, total	10 g
Carbohydrates	18 g	Fat, saturated	2 g
Fiber	3 g	Sodium	279 mg
Protein	26 g	Cholesterol	62 mg

Make-Ahead Southwestern Pork Stew (page 96)
Overleaf: Old-Fashioned Beef Stew (page 90)

Skillet Pork Stew

Tips
The apples in this super easy stew turn into a lovely sauce. Use pork shoulder, a leg steak, butt chops or a roast — whatever is on special.

This delicious pork stew is an excellent source of vitamins A and C, B vitamins and phosphorus, iron, magnesium and zinc.

1 lb	lean pork	500 g
2 tbsp	all-purpose flour	25 mL
¼ tsp	salt	1 mL
¼ tsp	pepper	1 mL
2 tbsp	vegetable oil (approx.)	25 mL
1	onion, coarsely chopped	1
1 cup	apple juice or water	250 mL
2 tsp	Dijon mustard	10 mL
2 tsp	vinegar	10 mL
½ tsp	dried thyme	2 mL
4	cloves garlic, halved	4
2	carrots, cut in 2-inch (5 cm) pieces	2
2	apples, peeled and quartered	2
5	small potatoes, quartered	4
1 cup	frozen peas	250 mL

1. Cut pork into 1-inch (2.5 cm) cubes. In bag, combine flour, salt and pepper; add pork and shake to coat. Set aside.

2. In large skillet, heat half of the oil over low heat; cook onion for 5 minutes. Transfer to bowl.

3. Heat remaining oil over medium-high heat; brown pork, in batches if necessary and adding more oil if needed. Add to bowl.

4. Pour apple juice into skillet; bring to boil, scraping up brown bits from bottom of pan. Stir in mustard, vinegar and thyme. Return pork and onion to skillet. Add garlic, carrots and apples; cover and bring to boil. Reduce heat and cook for 15 minutes, stirring occasionally.

5. Add potatoes; cook for 15 to 20 minutes or until meat and vegetables are tender. Stir in peas; cook for 5 minutes.

FOOD CHOICE VALUES PER SERVING

1½ ■ Starch Choices

2 ◢ Fruit & Vegetable Choices

3 ◑ Protein Choices

1 ▲ Fats & Oils Choice

NUTRIENT ANALYSIS PER SERVING			
Calories	424	Fat, total	14 g
Carbohydrates	47 g	Fat, saturated	3 g
Fiber	5 g	Sodium	250 mg
Protein	28 g	Cholesterol	68 mg

Slow cooker

Tip

Ghee is a type of clarified butter, highly valued in Indian cooking as it can be heated to a very high temperature. It is available in grocery stores specializing in Indian ingredients and will keep, refrigerated, for as long as a year.

Make ahead

This dish must be assembled the night before it is cooked as it needs to be marinated overnight. Follow preparation directions and refrigerate overnight. The next day, transfer to stoneware and cook as directed.

FOOD CHOICE VALUES PER SERVING

½ ◨ Fruit & Vegetable Choice

3½ ◨ Protein Choices

Pork Vindaloo

1 tbsp	cumin seeds	15 mL
2 tsp	coriander seeds	10 mL
1 tbsp	clarified butter or ghee (see Tip)	15 mL
1	onion, finely chopped	1
8	cloves garlic, minced	8
1 tbsp	minced gingerroot	15 mL
1	piece cinnamon stick, about 2 inches (5 cm)	1
6	whole cloves	6
½ tsp	salt	2 mL
2 tsp	mustard seeds	10 mL
¼ tsp	cayenne pepper	1 mL
2 lbs	stewing pork, cut into 1-inch (2.5-cm) cubes	1 kg
4	bay leaves	4
½ cup	red wine vinegar	125 mL

1. In a skillet, over medium heat, cook cumin and coriander seeds, stirring constantly, until they release their aroma and just begin to turn golden. Remove pan from heat and transfer seeds to a mortar or a cutting board. Using a pestle or a rolling pin, crush seeds coarsely. Set aside.

2. In a skillet, heat butter or ghee over medium heat. Add onion, garlic and gingerroot and cook for 1 minute. Add cumin and coriander seeds, cinnamon, cloves, salt, mustard seeds and cayenne and cook for 1 more minute. Remove from heat. Let cool.

3. Place pork in a mixing bowl. Add bay leaves and contents of pan. Add vinegar and stir to combine. Cover and marinate overnight in refrigerator. The next day, transfer to slow cooker stoneware, cover and cook on Low for 8 to 10 hours or on High for 4 to 5 hours, until pork is tender. Discard bay leaves, cinnamon stick and whole cloves.

NUTRIENT ANALYSIS PER SERVING			
Calories	181	Fat, total	6 g
Carbohydrates	4 g	Fat, saturated	2 g
Fiber	1 g	Sodium	225 mg
Protein	26 g	Cholesterol	82 mg

Deep baking dish,
measuring about 12 by
16 inches (30 by 40 cm)

Tips

Baked beans take many
forms around the world,
and cassoulet is the
version favored in the
well-fed northern regions
of France. There, any
number of fatty meats
(goose and/or pork fat,
for example) are mixed
with beans and baked
under an equally fatty
crust. Here we
"Mediterraneanize"
the original recipe, using
additional vegetables
and a lot less fat. Still,
this is a hefty and
lengthy dish that
requires cool weather,
a suitable occasion (to
justify the effort), and
a well-ventilated room.

This recipe is an
excellent source
of vitamin A, the
B vitamins, iron,
magnesium,
phosphorus and zinc.

FOOD CHOICE VALUES PER SERVING

2	■	Starch Choices
2	◨	Fruit & Vegetable Choices
3½	◎	Protein Choices
½	▲	Fats & Oils Choice
1	✦✦	Extra Choice

Cassoulet with Pork and Zucchini

1 tbsp	olive oil	15 mL
¼ tsp	salt, optional	1 mL
¼ tsp	freshly ground black pepper	1 mL
1 lb	pork tenderloin, cut into 1-inch (2.5 cm) cubes	500 g
1 tbsp	finely chopped garlic	15 mL
1 tbsp	olive oil	15 mL
½ tsp	salt, optional	2 mL
½ tsp	freshly ground black pepper	2 mL
1 cup	finely diced onions	250 mL
2	medium leeks, trimmed, washed and finely chopped (about 3 cups/750 mL)	2
2	stalks celery with leaves, finely chopped	2
Half	green pepper, finely diced	Half
1	large carrot, scraped and finely diced (about 4 oz/125 g)	1
8 oz	mushrooms, trimmed and quartered	250 g
1 lb	tomatoes, peeled and finely chopped (about 2 cups/500 mL) or canned tomatoes	500 g
1 tbsp	tomato paste, diluted in 1 cup (250 mL) water	15 mL
1 tsp	red wine vinegar	5 mL
1 tsp	dried basil	5 mL
1 tsp	dried oregano	5 mL
2 cups	cooked white kidney beans or 1 can (19 oz/540 mL), rinsed and drained	500 mL
2 cups	cooked red Romano beans or 1 can (19 oz/540 mL), rinsed and drained	500 mL

continued on page 101

NUTRIENT ANALYSIS PER SERVING

Calories	476	Fat, total	12 g
Carbohydrates	57 g	Fat, saturated	2 g
Fiber	5 g	Sodium	383 mg
Protein	31 g	Cholesterol	87 mg

1	medium zucchini cut into	1
	¼-inch (5 mm) rounds	
	(about 8 oz/250 g)	
2 cups	low-sodium chicken stock	500 mL

TOPPING

2 cups	breadcrumbs	500 mL
1 tbsp	finely chopped garlic	15 mL
½ tsp	ground allspice	2 mL
2	eggs, beaten	2
2 tbsp	olive oil	25 mL
1 cup	dry white vermouth	250 mL
	or white wine	
	Few sprigs fresh parsley, chopped	

1. In a large nonstick frying pan, heat 1 tbsp (15 mL) olive oil, optional ¼ tsp (1 mL) salt and pepper over high heat for 30 seconds. Add pork and stir-fry for 2 minutes, turning meat often so that all the pieces are thoroughly browned. Add garlic and stir-fry 1 more minute. Transfer contents of the frying pan to a large saucepan.

2. Return the frying pan to high heat. Add 1 tbsp (15 mL) olive oil, optional ½ tsp (2 mL) salt and pepper; heat for 30 seconds. Add onions, leeks, celery, green pepper, carrot and mushrooms; cook, stirring, for 4 minutes or until the vegetables are softened and a little oily. Transfer vegetables to saucepan with meat.

3. Stir in tomatoes, diluted tomato paste, vinegar, dried basil and oregano. Bring to a boil, cover tightly, reduce heat to medium-low and cook for 25 to 30 minutes or until the meat is cooked through. Remove from heat.

4. Preheat oven to 375°F (190°C). Add white kidney beans, red Romano beans, zucchini and chicken stock to the stew. Gently fold to mix everything thoroughly. Transfer this mixture to baking dish. Spread mixture over bottom of dish, making a layer about 1½ inches (4 cm) deep.

continued on page 102

5. *Topping:* In a bowl stir together the breadcrumbs, garlic and allspice until combined. In a small bowl, combine the eggs, olive oil and vermouth. Add this liquid to the breadcrumbs and stir to mix until combined (it'll be wet and lumpy).

6. As evenly as possible, spread this topping over the stew. Bake uncovered for 30 minutes. Remove from oven and press the topping (which will have browned a little) just into the stew, but leaving it still on top. Put back in the oven and bake another 30 minutes until the topping is nicely crusted and the stew is bubbling underneath.

7. Remove from oven and let rest 10 minutes. Portion onto plates, keeping breadcrumbs on top; garnish with chopped parsley and serve immediately.

Leek and Halibut Ragout

Tips

Don't overcook the vegetables in this main course dish; they should still retain their bright color and texture.

Saffron makes this stew special; you can, however, eliminate the saffron and substitute chopped fresh dill for the parsley.

2 tbsp	olive oil	25 mL
2	medium leeks, white and light green part only, chopped	2
2	cloves garlic, finely chopped	2
2 tbsp	all-purpose flour	25 mL
2 ½ cups	fish stock (see recipe, page 29) or chicken stock	625 mL
½ cup	white wine or additional stock	125 mL
¼ tsp	saffron threads, crushed	1 mL
2 cups	diced peeled potatoes	500 mL
2	medium carrots, peeled and diagonally sliced	2
2	small zucchini, halved lengthwise and sliced	2
1	small sweet red pepper, diced	1
1 ½ lbs	halibut, trimmed and cut into 1-inch (2.5 cm) cubes	750 g
	Salt and pepper	
¼ cup	chopped fresh parsley	50 mL

1. In a large saucepan, heat oil over medium heat; add leeks and garlic; cook, stirring often, for 5 minutes or until tender. (Do not let leeks brown.)

2. Stir in flour; add stock, wine and saffron. Bring to a boil, stirring, until thickened. Add potatoes and carrots; reduce heat to medium-low and simmer, covered, for 15 minutes. Stir in zucchini and red pepper; cook 5 minutes more or until vegetables are just tender.

3. Add halibut; cook for 3 to 5 minutes more or until fish is opaque. Adjust seasoning with salt and pepper to taste. Sprinkle with parsley; ladle into warmed wide shallow bowls.

FOOD CHOICE VALUES PER SERVING

1 ■ Starch Choice

1 ◗ Fruit & Vegetable Choice

3½ ◙ Protein Choices

NUTRIENT ANALYSIS PER SERVING

Calories	310	Fat, total	8 g
Carbohydrates	27 g	Fat, saturated	1 g
Fiber	3 g	Sodium	388 mg
Protein	29 g	Cholesterol	36 mg

Tips

To store gingerroot,
peel it, place in glass jar
and add white wine or
sherry to cover. As an
added bonus, you can
use the ginger-infused
wine or sherry to flavor
other fish or chicken
dishes, or stir-fries.

One of the best uses
for the microwave in my
kitchen is for quickly
cooking fish such as this
salmon. Arrange fish and
sauce in a shallow baking
dish and cover with
microwave-safe plastic
wrap; turn back one
corner to vent.
Microwave at Medium
for 4 minutes. Turn fish
over and re-cover;
microwave at Medium
for 3 to 5 minutes more
or until salmon
turns opaque.

This fish dish is
also great to cook
on the barbecue.

Salmon with Lemon-Ginger Sauce

MARINADE

2	green onions	2
1 ½ tsp	minced fresh gingerroot	7 mL
1	clove garlic, minced	1
2 tbsp	low-sodium soya sauce	25 mL
1 tbsp	fresh lemon juice	15 mL
1 tsp	grated lemon rind	5 mL
1 tsp	granulated sugar	5 mL
1 tsp	sesame oil	5 mL
4	salmon fillets, 5 oz (150 g) each	4

1. *Marinade:* Chop green onions; set aside chopped green tops for garnish. In a bowl combine white part of onions, gingerroot, garlic, soya sauce, lemon juice and rind, sugar and sesame oil.

2. Place salmon fillets in a single layer in a shallow baking dish. Pour marinade over; let stand at room temperature for 15 minutes or in the refrigerator for up to 1 hour.

3. Bake, uncovered, in preheated oven for 13 to 15 minutes or until salmon turns opaque. Arrange on serving plates, spoon sauce over and sprinkle with green onion tops.

NUTRIENT ANALYSIS PER SERVING

Calories	237	Fat, total	11 g
Carbohydrates	3 g	Fat, saturated	2 g
Fiber	0 g	Sodium	293 mg
Protein	31 g	Cholesterol	83 mg

Tips

Potato slices replace the usual bread in this homey and economical main dish.

Canned salmon with the bones makes this dish an excellent source of calcium. It is also an excellent source of vitamins A, D, B_6 and B_{12} as well as phosphorus, iron, magnesium and zinc.

Salmon and Potato Strata

1	can (7$\frac{1}{2}$ oz/213 g) red sockeye salmon	1
2	stalks celery, sliced	2
1	onion, chopped	1
4	eggs	4
1$\frac{1}{3}$ cups	milk	325 mL
$\frac{3}{4}$ tsp	paprika	4 mL
$\frac{3}{4}$ tsp	salt, optional	4 mL
$\frac{1}{2}$ tsp	pepper	2 mL
$\frac{1}{2}$ tsp	dried tarragon	2 mL
4	potatoes, peeled and thinly sliced	4
$\frac{1}{2}$ cup	dry bread crumbs	125 mL
$\frac{1}{4}$ cup	chopped fresh parsley	50 mL
2 tbsp	margarine or butter, cut in bits	25 mL

1. In large bowl, mash salmon with juices and bones; stir in celery, onion, eggs, milk, paprika, optional $\frac{1}{2}$ tsp (2 mL) salt, pepper and tarragon until well mixed.

2. In greased 8-cup (2 L) casserole, arrange half of the potato slices; sprinkle with optional remaining salt. Pour salmon mixture over top; layer with remaining potato slices.

3. Stir together crumbs and parsley, sprinkle on potatoes. Dot with butter. Bake, uncovered, in 350°F (180°C) oven for 1 hour and 15 minutes or until potatoes are tender.

FOOD CHOICE VALUES PER SERVING

2 ■ Starch Choices

$\frac{1}{2}$ ◢ Fruit & Vegetable Choice

2$\frac{1}{2}$ ◐ Protein Choices

2 ▲ Fats & Oils Choices

NUTRIENT ANALYSIS PER SERVING			
Calories	397	Fat, total	17 g
Carbohydrates	38 g	Fat, saturated	4 g
Fiber	3 g	Sodium	500 mg
Protein	23 g	Cholesterol	230 mg

Preheat broiler

Baking dish sprayed
with vegetable spray

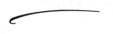

Tips

After broiling pepper,
put in small bowl and
cover tightly with plastic
wrap; this allows the skin
to be removed easily.

The fresh pepper can
be replaced with 4 oz
(125 g) sweet pepper
packed in water in a jar.

Roasted corn gives an
exceptional flavor in this
recipe. Either barbecue
or broil until just cooked
and charred, along with
pepper. Remove kernels
with a sharp knife.

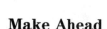

Make Ahead

Prepare salsa earlier in
the day and refrigerate.

Fish Fillets with Corn and Red Pepper Salsa

SALSA

1	large red pepper	1
1½ cups	corn kernels	375 mL
⅓ cup	chopped red onions	75 mL
¼ cup	chopped fresh coriander	50 mL
2 tbsp	fresh lime or lemon juice	25 mL
3 tsp	olive oil	15 mL
2 tsp	minced garlic	7 mL
1 lb	fish fillets	500 g

1. *Salsa:* Broil red pepper for 15 to 20 minutes, turning occasionally, until charred on all sides. Remove pepper and set oven at 425°F (220°C). When pepper is cool, remove skin, seeds and stem. Chop and put in small bowl along with corn, onions, coriander, lime juice, 2 tsp (10 mL) of olive oil and 1 tsp (5 mL) of the garlic; mix well.

2. Put fish in single layer in prepared baking dish and brush with remaining 1 tsp (5 mL) garlic and 1 tsp (5 mL) oil. Bake uncovered for 10 minutes per inch (2.5 cm) thickness of fish or until fish flakes easily when pierced with a fork. Serve with salsa.

FOOD CHOICE VALUES PER SERVING

1   ■ Starch Choice

½   ◨ Fruit & Vegetable Choice

3   ◐ Protein Choices

NUTRIENT ANALYSIS PER SERVING			
Calories	218	Fat, total	5 g
Carbohydrates	21 g	Fat, saturated	1 g
Fiber	3 g	Sodium	87 mg
Protein	24 g	Cholesterol	65 mg

Vegetables and Other Sides

Tips
Try making this dish with green beans. Trim and cut into 1½-inch (4 cm) lengths and cook in boiling water for about 5 minutes or until tender-crisp.

Asparagus makes this recipe an excellent source of folic acid.

Asparagus with Parmesan and Toasted Almonds

1½ lbs	asparagus	750 g
¼ cup	sliced blanched almonds	50 mL
2 tbsp	margarine or butter	25 mL
2	cloves garlic, finely chopped	2
¼ cup	freshly grated Parmesan cheese	50 mL
	Salt and freshly ground black pepper	

1. Snap off asparagus ends; cut spears on the diagonal into 2-inch (5 cm) lengths. In a large nonstick skillet, bring ½ cup (125 mL) water to a boil; cook asparagus for 2 minutes (start timing when water returns to a boil) or until just tender-crisp. Run under cold water to chill; drain and reserve.

2. Dry the skillet and place over medium heat. Add almonds and toast, stirring often, for 2 to 3 minutes or until golden. Remove and reserve.

3. Increase heat to medium-high. Add butter to skillet; cook asparagus and garlic, stirring, for 4 minutes or until asparagus is just tender.

4. Sprinkle with Parmesan; season with salt and pepper. Transfer to serving bowl; top with almonds.

FOOD CHOICE VALUES PER SERVING

½ ◖ Fruit & Vegetable Choice

½ ◉ Protein Choice

1 ▲ Fats & Oils Choice

NUTRIENT ANALYSIS PER SERVING			
Calories	107	Fat, total	8 g
Carbohydrates	7 g	Fat, saturated	4 g
Fiber	2 g	Sodium	113 mg
Protein	5 g	Cholesterol	14 mg

Tips

Most often made with rice, this barley risotto is a pleasant alternative to the traditional.

The peppers in this dish contribute almost 2 days' vitamin C in one serving.

Barley Risotto with Grilled Peppers

1	medium red bell pepper	1
1	medium yellow bell pepper	1
3½ to 4 cups	vegetable stock (see recipe, page 28) or chicken stock	875 mL to 1 L
1 cup	pearl barley	250 mL
1 cup	chopped onions	250 mL
2 tsp	minced garlic	10 mL
3 tbsp	grated low-fat Parmesan cheese	45 mL
¼ tsp	freshly ground black pepper	1 mL

1. Place red pepper and yellow pepper on baking sheet. Cook under preheated broiler, turning occasionally, for 20 minutes or until charred on all sides; remove from oven. When cool enough to handle, peel, stem and core peppers. Cut into chunks; set aside.

2. In a saucepan over medium-high heat, combine 2 cups (500 mL) stock with barley. Bring to a boil; reduce heat to low. Cook, stirring occasionally, for 30 minutes or until tender but firm. Set aside.

3. In a large nonstick frying pan sprayed with vegetable spray, cook onions and garlic over medium-high heat for 4 minutes or until softened. Add 1½ cups (375 mL) remaining stock; bring to a boil. Add cooked barley and roasted peppers; bring to a boil, stirring often. Reduce heat to medium-low; cook, stirring often, for 10 minutes or until barley is creamy. Add extra stock as needed. Add Parmesan cheese and pepper. Serve immediately.

FOOD CHOICE VALUES PER SERVING

2½ ▣ Starch Choices

1 ◪ Fruit & Vegetable Choice

NUTRIENT ANALYSIS PER SERVING

Calories	231	Fat, total	1 g
Carbohydrates	51 g	Fat, saturated	0 g
Fiber	6 g	Sodium	46 mg
Protein	7 g	Cholesterol	0 mg

Tip
This recipe makes an
excellent lunch base.
Round out the meal by
adding any missing
choices for your meal
plan, such as additional
protein, some whole
grain bread and a
milk serving.

Barley with Tomato, Red Onion, Goat Cheese and Basil

3 cups	vegetable stock (see recipe, page 28) or chicken stock	750 mL
3/4 cup	pearl barley	175 mL
3 cups	chopped ripe plum tomatoes	750 mL
1 cup	chopped red onions	250 mL
3/4 cup	chopped fresh basil (or 1 tsp/5 mL dried)	175 mL
2 oz	goat cheese, crumbled	50 g

DRESSING

1 tbsp	olive oil	15 mL
1 tbsp	fresh lemon juice	15 mL
1 tbsp	balsamic vinegar	15 mL
1 tsp	minced garlic	5 mL

1. In a saucepan over medium-high heat, bring stock to a boil. Add barley; reduce heat to medium-low. Cook, covered, for 45 minutes or until tender and liquid is absorbed. Transfer to a large serving bowl. Add tomatoes, red onions, basil and goat cheese; toss well.

2. *Dressing:* In a bowl combine olive oil, lemon juice, balsamic vinegar and garlic. Pour over barley mixture; toss to coat well. Serve warm or at room temperature.

FOOD CHOICE VALUES PER SERVING

1½ ■ Starch Choices

1½ ◢ Fruit & Vegetable Choices

½ ◉ Protein Choice

1 ▲ Fats & Oils Choice

NUTRIENT ANALYSIS PER SERVING

Calories	267	Fat, total	8 g
Carbohydrates	44 g	Fat, saturated	3 g
Fiber	6 g	Sodium	102 mg
Protein	9 g	Cholesterol	7 mg

Tips

The simple addition of cashews and red onions to this dish transforms ordinary green beans into a formidable companion to any gourmet main course.

Both the cashews and the oil contribute fat to this delicious dish. As with most plant sources of ▲ Fats & Oils, the majority of fat supplied is monounsaturated. Nutrient recommendations suggest most of our fat (80%) come from these sources.

Green Beans with Cashews

1 lb	green beans, trimmed	500 g
2 tbsp	olive oil	25 mL
1/2 cup	slivered red onions	125 mL
1/3 cup	raw cashews	75 mL
1/4 tsp	salt	1 mL
1/4 tsp	black pepper	1 mL
	Few sprigs fresh parsley, chopped	

1. Blanch green beans in a pot of boiling water for 5 minutes. Drain and immediately refresh in a bowl of ice-cold water. Drain and set aside.

2. In a large frying pan heat olive oil over medium-high heat for 30 seconds. Add onions, cashews, salt and pepper and stir-fry for 2 to 3 minutes, until the onions are softened. Add cooked green beans, raise heat to high, and stir-fry actively for 2 to 3 minutes, until the beans feel hot to the touch. (Take care that you don't burn any cashews in the process.) Transfer to a serving plate and garnish with chopped parsley. Serve immediately.

FOOD CHOICE VALUES PER SERVING

1	● Fruit & Vegetable Choice
1/2	● Protein Choice
2	▲ Fats & Oils Choices
1	●● Extra Choice

NUTRIENT ANALYSIS PER SERVING			
Calories	172	Fat, total	12 g
Carbohydrates	14 g	Fat, saturated	2 g
Fiber	3 g	Sodium	215 mg
Protein	4 g	Cholesterol	0 mg

Preheat oven to
350°F (180°C)

10-cup (2.5 L) shallow
baking dish, greased

Tips

To make fresh bread
crumbs, process 2 thick
slices crusty bread in a
food processor until fine.

This recipe is an
excellent source of
vitamin C, magnesium
and folic acid.

Baked White Beans with Garlic Crumb Crust

3 tbsp	olive oil	45 mL
2 cups	chopped Spanish onion	500 mL
3	cloves garlic, finely chopped	3
2 tbsp	balsamic vinegar	25 mL
5	tomatoes, seeded and diced	5
1 tbsp	chopped fresh thyme or 1 tsp (5 mL) dried thyme leaves	15 mL
1	large bay leaf	1
	Salt and freshly ground black pepper	
2	zucchini, halved lengthwise, thickly sliced	2
1	red bell pepper, diced	1
1	yellow bell pepper, diced	1
2	cans (each 19 oz/ 540 mL) white kidney beans, drained and rinsed	2

GARLIC CRUMB CRUST

1 1/2 cups	soft fresh bread crumbs (see Tip)	375 mL
1/4 cup	chopped fresh parsley	50 mL
2	cloves garlic, minced	2
2 tbsp	olive oil	25 mL

1. In a Dutch oven or large saucepan, heat oil over medium heat. Cook onions and garlic, stirring often, for 5 minutes or until softened. Add balsamic vinegar and cook until evaporated. Add tomatoes, thyme and bay leaf; season with salt and pepper. Bring to boil. Reduce heat, cover and simmer for 20 minutes.

2. Add zucchini and peppers; cook for 5 to 7 minutes or until vegetables are tender-crisp. Gently stir in beans.

continued on page 113

FOOD CHOICE VALUES PER SERVING

1   ■ Starch Choice

1   ◢ Fruit & Vegetable Choice

1   ◉ Protein Choice

1 1/2   ▲ Fats & Oils Choices

NUTRIENT ANALYSIS PER SERVING			
Calories	261	Fat, total	10 g
Carbohydrates	37 g	Fat, saturated	1 g
Fiber	11 g	Sodium	475 mg
Protein	10 g	Cholesterol	0 mg

3. Spoon mixture into prepared baking dish. (Can be prepared up to this point, covered and refrigerated for up to one day.)

4. *Garlic Crumb Crust:* In a bowl, combine bread crumbs, parsley and garlic. Drizzle with olive oil and toss to coat. Sprinkle crumb topping over beans; bake for 35 to 45 minutes or until bubbly and top is golden.

Bean Salad with Mustard-Dill Dressing

1 lb	green beans	500 g
1	can (19 oz/540 mL) chickpeas, rinsed and drained	1
⅓ cup	chopped red onions	75 mL
2 tbsp	finely chopped fresh dill	25 mL
2 tbsp	olive oil	25 mL
2 tbsp	red wine vinegar	25 mL
1 tbsp	Dijon mustard	15 mL
1 tbsp	granulated sugar	15 mL
¼ tsp	salt	1 mL
¼ tsp	pepper	1 mL

1. Trim ends of beans; cut into 1-inch (2.5 cm) lengths. In a large pot of boiling salted water, cook beans for 3 to 5 minutes (count from time water returns to boil) or until tender-crisp. Drain; rinse under cold water to chill. Drain well.

2. In a serving bowl, combine green beans, chickpeas, onions and dill.

3. In a small bowl, whisk together oil, vinegar, mustard, sugar, salt and pepper until smooth.

4. Pour over beans and toss well. Refrigerate until serving.

NUTRIENT ANALYSIS PER SERVING			
Calories	219	Fat, total	7 g
Carbohydrates	32 g	Fat, saturated	1 g
Fiber	5 g	Sodium	324 mg
Protein	9 g	Cholesterol	0 mg

Moors and Christians

1	roasted red bell pepper, finely chopped	1
1 tbsp	vegetable oil	15 mL
2	medium onions, finely chopped	2
4	large cloves garlic, minced	4
2 tsp	dried oregano leaves	10 mL
2 tsp	cumin seeds	10 mL
1	medium tomato, peeled, seeded and chopped	1
1	can (19 oz/540 mL) black beans, rinsed and drained, or 1 cup (250 mL) dried black beans, cooked and drained	1
½ cup	condensed chicken broth (undiluted)	125 mL
2 cups	long-grain rice	500 mL
1	green bell pepper, finely chopped	1
2 tbsp	lemon or lime juice	25 mL
¼ cup	finely chopped cilantro	50 mL
4	green onions, white part only, finely chopped	4

Tips

Although there are several different versions of how this classic Cuban dish got its name, all lead back to the eighth century when Spain was invaded by their enemies, the Moors.

This dish is also delicious cold and makes a nice addition to a buffet as a rice salad.

An excellent source of vitamin C.

1. In a skillet, heat oil over medium heat. Add onion and cook until soft. Add garlic, oregano and cumin seeds and cook for 1 minute. Stirring, add roasted red pepper, tomato, beans and chicken broth and bring to a boil. Transfer to slow cooker stoneware.

2. Cover and cook on Low for 8 to 10 hours or on High for 4 to 5 hours.

3. When bean mixture is cooked, make rice. In a heavy pot with a tight-fitting lid, combine rice with 4 cups (1 L) water. Cover, bring to a rapid boil, then turn off the heat, leaving the pot on the warm element. Do not lift the lid or move the pot until rice is ready, which will take about 20 minutes.

continued on page 115

NUTRIENT ANALYSIS PER SERVING			
Calories	247	Fat, total	3 g
Carbohydrates	49 g	Fat, saturated	0 g
Fiber	3 g	Sodium	101 mg
Protein	7 g	Cholesterol	0 mg

4. Meanwhile, add green pepper to contents of slow cooker and stir well. Cover and cook on High for 20 to 30 minutes, until pepper is tender.

5. Stir cooked rice into slow cooker. Add lemon or lime juice, cilantro and green onions and stir to combine thoroughly. Serve hot as a main course or cold as a salad.

Cumin Beets

SERVES 6

Slow cooker

Tip
Peeling the beets before they are cooked ensures that all the delicious cooking juices end up on your plate.

Make ahead
This dish can be assembled the night before it is cooked. Complete Step 1, add beets to mixture and refrigerate overnight. The next day, continue cooking as directed in Step 2.

1 tbsp	vegetable oil	15 mL
1	onion, finely chopped	1
3	cloves garlic, minced	3
1 tsp	cumin seeds	5 mL
1 tsp	salt	5 mL
1/2 tsp	black pepper	2 mL
2	medium tomatoes, peeled and coarsely chopped	2
1 cup	water	250 mL
1 lb	beets, peeled and used whole, if small, or sliced thinly (see Tip)	500 g

1. In a skillet, heat oil over medium-high heat. Add onion and cook, stirring, until softened. Stir in garlic, cumin, salt and pepper and cook for 1 minute. Add tomatoes and water and bring to a boil.

2. Place beets in slow cooker stoneware and pour tomato mixture over them. Cover and cook on Low for 8 to 10 hours or on High for 4 to 5 hours, until beets are tender.

FOOD CHOICE VALUES PER SERVING

1 ◗ Fruit & Vegetable Choice

1/2 ▲ Fats & Oils Choice

NUTRIENT ANALYSIS PER SERVING			
Calories	70	Fat, total	3 g
Carbohydrates	11 g	Fat, saturated	0 g
Fiber	2 g	Sodium	426 mg
Protein	2 g	Cholesterol	0 mg

Pasta and Bean Salad with Creamy Basil Dressing

DRESSING

1 1/2 cups	tightly packed fresh basil leaves	375 mL
3 tbsp	grated low-fat Parmesan cheese	45 mL
2 tbsp	toasted pine nuts	25 mL
1 1/2 tsp	minced garlic	7 mL
1/3 cup	low-fat yogurt	75 mL
3 tbsp	fresh lemon juice	45 mL
3 tbsp	light mayonnaise	45 mL
3 tbsp	water	45 mL
1 tbsp	olive oil	15 mL
1/4 tsp	freshly ground black pepper	1 mL

SALAD

12 oz	medium shell pasta	375 g
3/4 cup	canned black beans, rinsed and drained	175 mL
3/4 cup	canned chickpeas, rinsed and drained	175 mL
3/4 cup	canned red kidney beans, rinsed and drained	175 mL
3/4 cup	diced red onions	175 mL
1/2 cup	shredded carrots	125 mL
2 cups	diced ripe plum tomatoes	500 mL

1. *Dressing:* In a food processor or blender, combine basil, Parmesan cheese, pine nuts and garlic; process until finely chopped. Add yogurt, lemon juice, mayonnaise, water, olive oil and pepper; purée until smooth. Set aside.

continued on page 117

NUTRIENT ANALYSIS PER SERVING			
Calories	289	Fat, total	7 g
Carbohydrates	49 g	Fat, saturated	1 g
Fiber	4 g	Sodium	64 mg
Protein	10 g	Cholesterol	0 mg

2. *Salad:* In a large pot of boiling water, cook pasta for 8 to 10 minutes or until tender but firm; drain. Rinse under cold running water; drain.

3. In a serving bowl, combine pasta, black beans, chickpeas, kidney beans, red onions, carrots and plum tomatoes. Pour dressing over salad; toss to coat well. Serve immediately.

Jalapeno Broccoli

Tips
This salad can be served immediately or it can wait up to 2 hours, covered and unrefrigerated.

This side dish is an excellent source of vitamin A and C and folic acid.

If you use the salt here, the sodium is 644 mg per serving.

1 tsp	salt, optional	5 mL
1	head broccoli, trimmed and separated into spears	1
1 tbsp	balsamic vinegar	15 mL
2-3 tbsp	olive oil	25-45 mL
2	fresh jalapeno peppers, thinly sliced (with or without seeds, depending on desired hotness)	2
1/4 cup	toasted pine nuts	50 mL
	Few sprigs fresh coriander or parsley, chopped	

1. Bring a pot of water to the boil and add optional salt. Add the broccoli spears and boil over high heat for 3 to 5 minutes (depending on desired tenderness). Drain and transfer broccoli to bowl of ice cold water for 30 seconds. Drain and lay out the cooked spears decoratively on a presentation plate. Drizzle evenly with balsamic vinegar.

2. In a small frying pan, heat olive oil over medium heat for 30 seconds. Add sliced jalapeno peppers (with seeds, if using) and stir-fry for 2 to 3 minutes until softened. Take peppers with all the oil from the pan, and distribute evenly over the broccoli. Garnish with pine nuts and herbs.

FOOD CHOICE VALUES PER SERVING

1   ◗   Fruit & Vegetable Choice

1   ◙   Protein Choice

1   ▲   Fats & Oils Choice

NUTRIENT ANALYSIS PER SERVING			
Calories	142	Fat, total	9 g
Carbohydrates	14 g	Fat, saturated	1 g
Fiber	6 g	Sodium	206 mg
Protein	8 g	Cholesterol	0 mg

While North American tastes are generally restricted to broccoli florets, Asian cooking also uses broccoli stalks extensively. So don't throw them away — trim the woody bottoms and peel the stalks using a paring knife; then cut the tender, mild interior into slices or strips.

Broccoli and peppers are a winning combination, providing excellent sources of vitamins A and C and folic acid.

Orange Broccoli with Red Pepper

1/3 cup	orange juice	75 mL
1/2 tsp	cornstarch	2 mL
1 tbsp	olive oil	15 mL
4 cups	small broccoli florets and stalks, cut into 1 1/2- by 1/2-inch (4 by 1 cm) lengths	1 L
1	sweet red pepper, cut into 2- by 1/2-inch (5 by 1 cm) strips	1
1	clove garlic, minced	1
1 tsp	grated orange rind	5 mL
1/4 tsp	salt	1 mL
1/4 tsp	pepper	1 mL

1. In a glass measuring cup, stir together orange juice and cornstarch until smooth; reserve.

2. Heat oil in a large nonstick skillet over high heat. Add broccoli, red pepper and garlic; cook, stirring, for 2 minutes.

3. Add orange juice mixture; cover and cook 1 to 2 minutes or until vegetables are tender-crisp. Sprinkle with orange rind; season with salt and pepper. Serve immediately.

FOOD CHOICE VALUES PER SERVING

1/2 ■ Starch Choice

1/2 ◑ Protein Choice

1/2 ▲ Fats & Oils Choice

1 ✦✦ Extra Choice

NUTRIENT ANALYSIS PER SERVING			
Calories	78	Fat, total	4 g
Carbohydrates	10 g	Fat, saturated	1 g
Fiber	3 g	Sodium	161 mg
Protein	3 g	Cholesterol	0 mg

Sweet-and-Spicy Cabbage

For a modern spin of an Oktoberfest dinner, spoon cabbage in center of serving plates and top with grilled sausages or smoked pork chops.

Honey provides 5 g carbohydrate, or the ½ ✳ Sugars Choice in this recipe. A sugar substitute can replace this and reduce the carbohydrate by 5 g, eliminating the ½ ✳ Sugars Choice.

1	large pear or apple	1
2 tbsp	vegetable oil	25 mL
½	red onion, cut into thin wedge strips	½
½ tsp	hot pepper flakes or to taste	2 mL
½	small Savoy cabbage, finely shredded	½
2 tbsp	rice vinegar	25 mL
1 tbsp	liquid honey	15 mL
	Salt	

1. Cut pear into quarters and core (not necessary to peel). Thinly slice, then cut slices in half.

2. In a large nonstick skillet, heat oil over high heat until almost smoking. Add pear, onion and hot pepper flakes; stir-fry for 1 minute. Add cabbage and stir-fry for 1 minute more or until wilted.

3. Stir in rice vinegar and honey; cook, stirring, for 30 seconds. Season with salt to taste; serve immediately.

FOOD CHOICE VALUES PER SERVING

1 ◖ Fruit & Vegetable Choice

½ ✳ Sugars Choice

1½ ▲ Fats & Oils Choices

NUTRIENT ANALYSIS PER SERVING			
Calories	125	Fat, total	7 g
Carbohydrates	17 g	Fat, saturated	1 g
Fiber	3 g	Sodium	16 mg
Protein	2 g	Cholesterol	0 mg

Cauliflower and Red Pepper

Tips

A colorful, emphatically dressed combination of lush red pepper and the oft-neglected cauliflower, this salad travels well on picnics in the summer, just as it helps to liven up a cozy dinner in winter.

This is an excellent source of vitamins A and C.

1	head cauliflower, florets only	1
2	red bell peppers, roasted, skinned and cut into thick strips	2
1/4 tsp	salt	1 mL
1/4 tsp	black pepper	1 mL
2 tbsp	lemon juice	25 mL
1 tbsp	Dijon mustard	15 mL
1 tsp	vegetable oil	5 mL
1 tsp	black mustard seeds	5 mL
1/2 tsp	turmeric	2 mL
1/2 tsp	whole coriander seeds	2 mL
2	cloves garlic	2
2 tbsp	olive oil	25 mL

1. Blanch cauliflower florets in a large saucepan of boiling water for 5 to 6 minutes, until just cooked. Drain, refresh in iced water, drain again and transfer to a bowl. Add red peppers to cauliflower. Sprinkle with salt and pepper and toss.

2. In a small bowl whisk together the lemon juice and Dijon mustard until blended. Set aside.

3. In a small frying pan heat vegetable oil over medium heat for 1 minute. Add mustard seeds, turmeric and coriander seeds, and stir-fry for 2 to 3 minutes, or until the seeds begin to pop. With a rubber spatula, scrape cooked spices from the pan into the lemon-mustard mixture. Squeeze garlic through a garlic press and add to the mixture. Add olive oil and whisk until the dressing has emulsified.

continued on page 121

FOOD CHOICE VALUES PER SERVING

1/2 ◖ Fruit & Vegetable Choice

1 ▲ Fats & Oils Choice

NUTRIENT ANALYSIS PER SERVING

Calories	83	Fat, total	6 g
Carbohydrates	7 g	Fat, saturated	1 g
Fiber	2 g	Sodium	142 mg
Protein	2 g	Cholesterol	0 mg

4. Add dressing to the cauliflower-red pepper mixture. Toss gently but thoroughly to dress all the pieces evenly. Transfer to a serving bowl, propping up the red pepper ribbons to properly accent the yellow-tinted cauliflower. This salad benefits greatly from a 1- or 2-hour wait, after which it should be served at room temperature.

SERVES 4

Tips
If doubling the recipe, glaze vegetables in a large nonstick skillet to evaporate the stock quickly.

Try this tasty treatment with a combination of blanched carrots, rutabaga and parsnip strips, too.

This recipe contains almost 3 days' supply of vitamin A.

Lemon-Glazed Baby Carrots

1 lb	peeled baby carrots	500 g
¼ cup	chicken stock or vegetable stock (see recipe, page 28)	50 mL
1 tbsp	margarine or butter	15 mL
1 tbsp	brown sugar	15 mL
1 tbsp	lemon juice	15 mL
½ tsp	grated lemon rind	2 mL
¼ tsp	salt	1 mL
	Pepper to taste	
1 tbsp	finely chopped fresh parsley or chives	15 mL

1. In a medium saucepan, cook carrots in boiling salted water for 5 to 7 minutes (start timing when water returns to a boil) or until just tender-crisp; drain and return to saucepan.

2. Add stock, butter, brown sugar, lemon juice and rind, salt and pepper. Cook, stirring often, 3 to 5 minutes or until liquid has evaporated and carrots are nicely glazed.

3. Sprinkle with parsley or chives and serve.

FOOD CHOICE VALUES PER SERVING

1	◢	Fruit & Vegetable Choice
½	▲	Fats & Oils Choice
1	◆◆	Extra Choice

NUTRIENT ANALYSIS PER SERVING			
Calories	91	Fat, total	3 g
Carbohydrates	15 g	Fat, saturated	2 g
Fiber	3 g	Sodium	251 mg
Protein	2 g	Cholesterol	8 mg

Couscous Salad with Basil and Pine Nuts

1 cup	low-sodium chicken stock or vegetable stock (see recipe, page 28)	250 mL
1 cup	couscous	250 mL
4	green onions, chopped	4
1	sweet red pepper, diced	1
1	medium zucchini, diced	1
¼ cup	raisins	50 mL
¼ cup	olive oil	50 mL
2 tbsp	red wine vinegar	25 mL
2 tbsp	orange juice	25 mL
1 tsp	grated orange rind	5 mL
1	large garlic clove, minced	1
½ tsp	salt, optional	2 mL
	Pepper to taste	
¼ cup	chopped fresh basil	50 mL
¼ cup	toasted pine nuts	50 mL

1. Place couscous in a large bowl; pour stock over. Cover with a dinner plate and let stand for 5 minutes. Fluff with a fork to break up any lumps. Let cool to room temperature. Add onions, pepper, zucchini and raisins.

2. In a small bowl, whisk together oil, vinegar, orange juice and rind, garlic, optional salt and pepper. Pour over salad; toss well. Just before serving, stir in basil and pine nuts. Serve salad at room temperature.

FOOD CHOICE VALUES PER SERVING

2½ ■ Starch Choices

1 ◗ Fruit & Vegetable Choice

½ ◔ Protein Choice

3½ ▲ Fats & Oils Choices

NUTRIENT ANALYSIS PER SERVING			
Calories	406	Fat, total	19 g
Carbohydrates	51 g	Fat, saturated	3 g
Fiber	5 g	Sodium	132 mg
Protein	11 g	Cholesterol	0 mg

Preheat oven to
425°F (220°C)

Baking sheet sprayed
with vegetable spray

Tips

Couscous has been a
staple of North African
cuisine for centuries. It
is made with coarsely
ground semolina — a
hard wheat flour used for
pasta. Couscous is loaded
with fiber, vitamins and
minerals. For extra
flavor, try cooking it with
stock or tomato sauce.
It's a wonderful
replacement for pasta,
rice or other grains.

These cakes make terrific
vegetarian burgers! Just
place in a pita lined with
lettuce, tomatoes and
onions. Drizzle with
sauce and serve.

Greek Couscous Cakes

1½ cups	vegetable stock (see recipe, page 28) or chicken stock	375 mL
1 cup	couscous	250 mL
½ cup	minced red bell peppers	125 mL
⅓ cup	minced green onions	75 mL
⅓ cup	minced red onions	75 mL
¼ cup	minced black olives	50 mL
1 tsp	minced garlic	5 mL
1 tsp	dried oregano	5 mL
1½ oz	light feta cheese, crumbled	40 g
2	large egg whites	2
1	large egg	1
2 tbsp	fresh lemon juice	25 mL

SAUCE

½ cup	low-fat sour cream	125 mL
2 tsp	chopped fresh dill (or ⅛ tsp/0.5 mL dried)	10 mL
1 tsp	fresh lemon juice	5 mL
¼ tsp	minced garlic	1 mL

1. In a saucepan over high heat, bring stock to a boil. Add couscous; remove from heat. Let stand, covered, for 5 minutes or until liquid is absorbed and grain is tender. Fluff with a fork; set aside to cool.

2. In a bowl combine cooled couscous, red peppers, green onions, red onions, black olives, garlic, oregano, feta cheese, egg whites, whole egg and lemon juice. Form each ⅓ cup (75 mL) mixture into a flat patty, squeezing together in your hands. Place patties on prepared baking sheet. Bake in preheated oven, turning at halfway point, for 20 minutes or until golden.

3. *Sauce:* In a bowl combine sour cream, dill, lemon juice and garlic. Serve warm patties with sauce.

**FOOD CHOICE VALUES
PER SERVING**

1½ ■ Starch Choices

½ ◨ Fruit & Vegetable
Choice

1 ◨ Protein Choice

NUTRIENT ANALYSIS PER SERVING			
Calories	192	Fat, total	4 g
Carbohydrates	30 g	Fat, saturated	1 g
Fiber	2 g	Sodium	98 mg
Protein	9 g	Cholesterol	39 mg

Vegetable Couscous

Tips
This easy, flavorful
dish combines couscous,
a North African pasta,
with a spicy vegetable
stew. Look for instant
couscous in the rice
section of most large
supermarkets or in
bulk-food stores.

This may be more
☑ Fruit & Vegetable
Choices than on your
plan. Carrots, parsnips,
turnips, tomatoes and
raisins all contribute.
Reducing the raisins to
¼ cup (50 mL) to
eliminate ½ ☑ Fruit
& Vegetable Choice.

This recipe is an
excellent source
of vitamin A, iron,
magnesium and
folic acid.

2 tbsp	vegetable oil	25 mL
1	onion, cut in 2-inch (5 cm) chunks	1
1 tbsp	minced fresh ginger	15 mL
½ tsp	paprika	2 mL
½ tsp	pepper	2 mL
½ tsp	turmeric	2 mL
½ tsp	ground cumin	2 mL
Pinch	cayenne	Pinch
1	clove garlic, minced	1
3	carrots, cut in 2-inch (5 cm) chunks	3
3	parsnips, cut in 2-inch (5 cm) chunks	3
2	small white turnips, peeled and cut in wedges	2
2	tomatoes, peeled and quartered	2
1	can (19 oz/540 mL) chick-peas, drained and rinsed	1
2½ cups	chicken or vegetable stock (see recipe, page 28)	625 mL
2 cups	sliced green beans	500 mL
½ cup	seedless raisins	125 mL
	Salt	
1 cup	couscous	250 mL

1. In large wide heavy saucepan, heat oil over medium heat; cook onion for 2 minutes. Add ginger, paprika, pepper, turmeric, cumin and cayenne; cook for 3 minutes, stirring often.

2. Add garlic, carrots, parsnips, turnips, tomatoes, chick-peas and stock; bring to boil. Reduce heat to low; simmer, covered, for 15 minutes or until vegetables are almost tender.

continued on page 125

NUTRIENT ANALYSIS PER SERVING			
Calories	344	Fat, total	6 g
Carbohydrates	62 g	Fat, saturated	1 g
Fiber	8 g	Sodium	292 mg
Protein	13 g	Cholesterol	0 mg

3. Add beans and raisins; cook, uncovered, for 10 minutes or until beans are tender-crisp and liquid has thickened slightly. Season with salt to taste. (Stew can be prepared to this point, cooled, covered and refrigerated for up to 1 day. In this case, just cook 5 minutes after adding beans. Reheat gently.)

4. Meanwhile, in medium saucepan, boil $1\frac{1}{2}$ cups (375 mL) water; add couscous and $\frac{1}{2}$ tsp (2 mL) salt. Remove from heat. Let stand, covered, for 5 minutes or until couscous is tender and water is absorbed; fluff with fork. Spoon onto large heated platter; make well in center. Spoon in vegetable mixture.

Tip

A proper risotto is made with Italian short-grain rice. As it cooks, it gives off the starch and the constant stirring results in a creamy, moist texture similar to porridge. Arborio rice is the most widely available short-grain variety; look for the word superfino on the package to ensure you are buying a superior grade. Vialone nano and carnaroli are two other types of short-grain Italian rice that make wonderful risotto. They are not quite as starchy as Arborio and require slightly less stock in cooking.

Wild Mushroom Risotto

5 cups	low-sodium chicken or vegetable stock (see recipe, page 28) (approx.)	1.25 L
2 tbsp	butter	25 mL
2 tbsp	olive oil	25 mL
1 lb	assorted mushrooms, such as cremini, shiitake and oyster, coarsely chopped	500 g
2	cloves garlic, minced	2
1 tbsp	chopped fresh thyme or 1 tsp (5 mL) dried	15 mL
1/4 tsp	freshly ground black pepper	1 mL
1	small onion, finely chopped	1
1 1/2 cups	short-grain rice, such as Arborio	375 mL
1/2 cup	white wine or stock	125 mL
1/3 cup	freshly grated Parmesan cheese	75 mL
	Salt	
2 tbsp	chopped fresh parsley	25 mL

1. In a large saucepan, bring stock to a boil; reduce heat to low and keep hot.

2. In a heavy-bottomed medium saucepan, heat 1 tbsp (15 mL) each oil and butter over medium heat. Add mushrooms, garlic, thyme and pepper; cook, stirring often, for 5 to 7 minutes or until tender. Remove and set aside.

3. Add remaining butter and oil to saucepan; cook onion, stirring, for 2 minutes or until softened. Add rice; stir for 1 minute. Add wine; stir until absorbed.

4. Add 1 cup (250 mL) hot stock; adjust heat to a simmer so stock bubbles and is absorbed slowly.

continued on page 127

FOOD CHOICE VALUES PER SERVING

2 1/2 ■ Starch Choices

1 ◢ Fruit & Vegetable Choice

1 ◗ Protein Choice

2 ▲ Fats & Oils Choices

NUTRIENT ANALYSIS PER SERVING			
Calories	352	Fat, total	12 g
Carbohydrates	47 g	Fat, saturated	5 g
Fiber	1 g	Sodium	550 mg
Protein	12 g	Cholesterol	15 mg

5. When absorbed, continue adding 1 cup (250 mL) stock at a time, stirring almost constantly, for 15 minutes. Add mushroom mixture; cook, stirring often, adding more stock when absorbed, until rice is just tender but slightly firm in the center. Mixture should be creamy; add more stock or water, if necessary. (Total cooking time will be 20 to 25 minutes.)

6. Add Parmesan cheese; adjust seasoning with salt and pepper to taste. Spoon into warm shallow serving bowls or onto plates. Sprinkle with parsley; serve immediately.

SERVES 6

Tip
Other nuts, such as skinned hazelnuts or unblanched almonds, can be substituted for the walnuts.

Mushroom Barley Pilaf

1 tbsp	margarine or butter	15 mL
2 cups	sliced mushrooms	500 mL
1	small onion, chopped	1
½ tsp	dried thyme or marjoram leaves	2 mL
1 cup	pearl barley, rinsed	250 mL
2½ cups	chicken or vegetable stock (see recipe, page 28) (approx.)	625 mL
⅓ cup	finely chopped walnuts or pecans	75 mL
¼ cup	freshly grated Parmesan cheese	50 mL
2 tbsp	chopped fresh parsley	25 mL
	Salt and freshly ground black pepper	

1. In a medium saucepan, heat butter over medium heat. Add mushrooms, onion and thyme; cook, stirring, for 5 minutes or until softened.

2. Stir in barley and stock; bring to a boil. Reduce heat, cover and simmer, stirring occasionally and adding more stock if necessary, for 30 minutes or until barley is tender.

3. Stir in walnuts, Parmesan and parsley; season with salt and pepper to taste.

FOOD CHOICE VALUES PER SERVING

1½ ▣ Starch Choices

½ ◪ Fruit & Vegetable Choice

½ ◓ Protein Choice

1½ ▲ Fats & Oils Choices

NUTRIENT ANALYSIS PER SERVING			
Calories	222	Fat, total	8 g
Carbohydrates	30 g	Fat, saturated	3 g
Fiber	3 g	Sodium	405 mg
Protein	9 g	Cholesterol	8 mg

Slow cooker

Tip

This is a great dish
to serve with roasted
poultry or meat. If your
guests like spice, pass
hot pepper sauce
at the table.

New Orleans Braised Onions

2 to 3	large Spanish onions	2 to 3
6 to 9	whole cloves	6 to 9
1/2 tsp	salt	2 mL
1/2 tsp	cracked black peppercorns	2 mL
Pinch	ground thyme	Pinch
	Grated zest and juice of 1 orange	
1/2 cup	condensed beef broth, undiluted	125 mL
	Finely chopped fresh parsley, optional	
	Hot pepper sauce, optional	

1. Stud onions with cloves. Place in slow cooker stoneware and sprinkle with salt, peppercorns, thyme and orange zest. Pour orange juice and beef broth over onions, cover and cook on Low for 8 hours or on High for 4 hours, until onions are tender.

2. Keep onions warm. In a saucepan over medium heat, reduce cooking liquid by half.

3. When ready to serve, cut onions into quarters. Place on a deep platter and cover with sauce. Sprinkle with parsley, if desired, and pass the hot pepper sauce, if desired.

FOOD CHOICE VALUES PER SERVING

1/2 🍃 Fruit & Vegetable Choice

NUTRIENT ANALYSIS PER SERVING			
Calories	20	Fat, total	0 g
Carbohydrates	4 g	Fat, saturated	0 g
Fiber	1 g	Sodium	188 mg
Protein	1 g	Cholesterol	0 mg

Asparagus with Parmesan and Toasted Almonds (page 108)
Overleaf: *Green Beans with Cashews (page 111)*

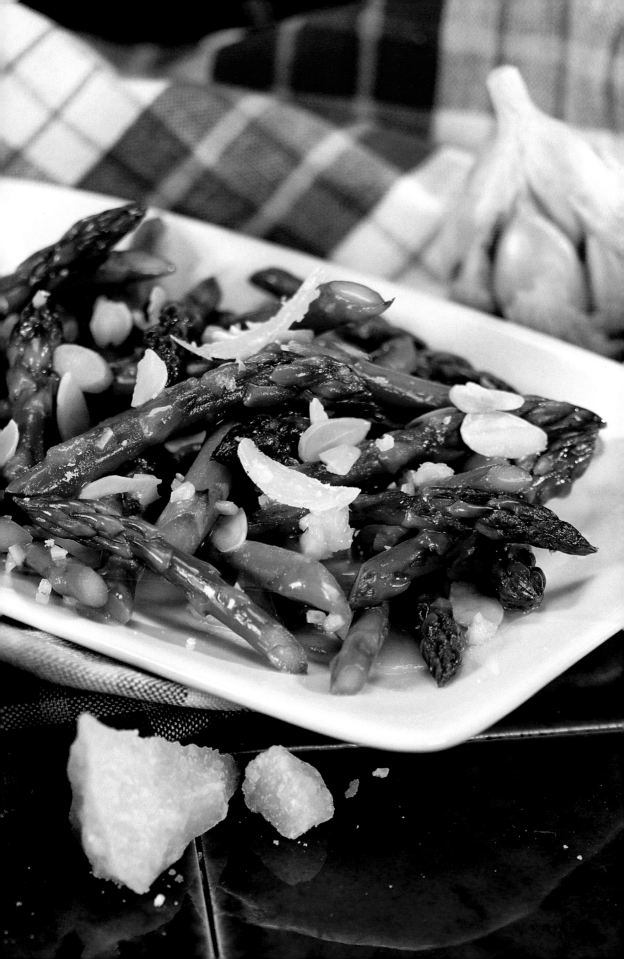

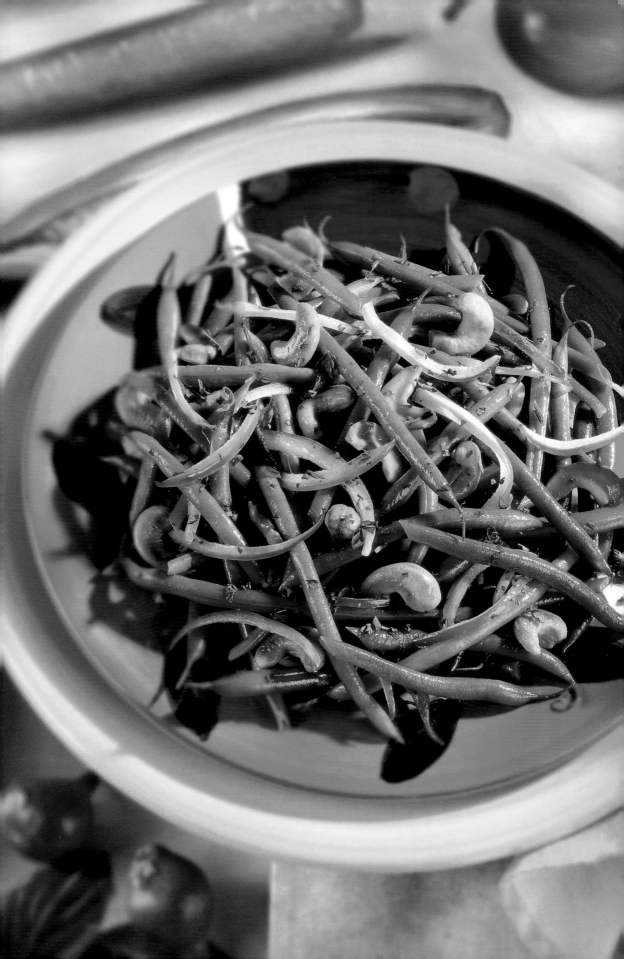

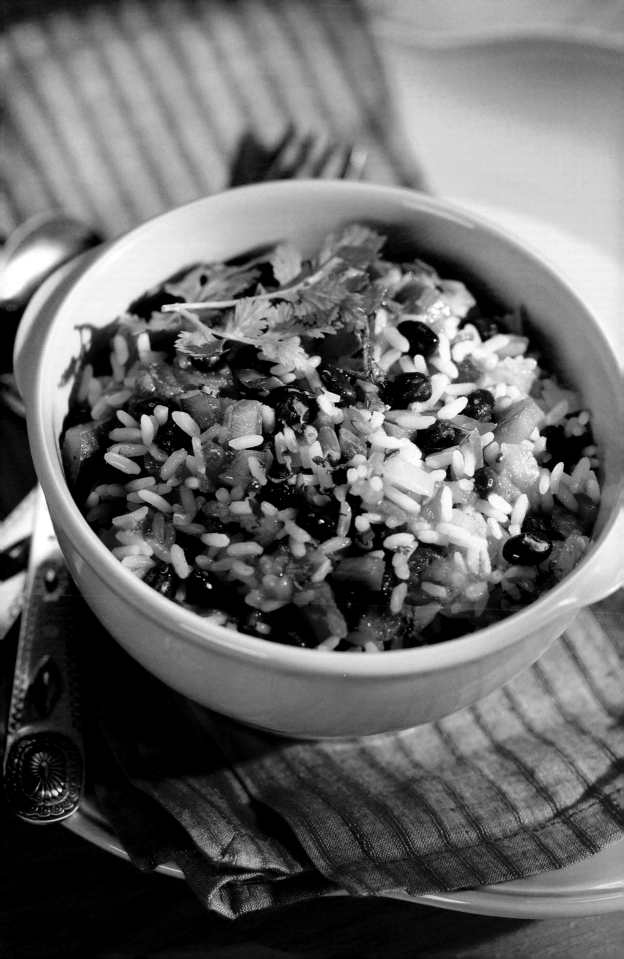

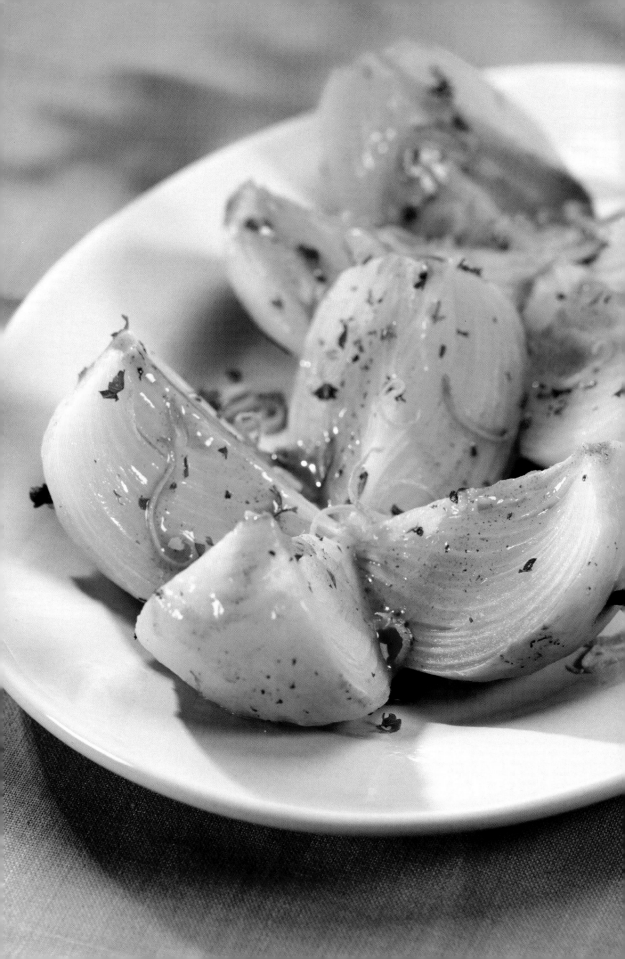

Slow cooker

Tip
Use your favorite hot sauce, such as Tabasco, Louisiana Hot Sauce, Piri Piri, or try other more exotic brands to vary the flavors in this recipe.

Peppery Red Onions

4	large red onions, quartered	4
1 tbsp	extra-virgin olive oil	15 mL
1 tsp	dried oregano leaves	5 mL
1/4 cup	water or chicken or vegetable stock (see recipe, page 28)	50 mL
	Salt and pepper, to taste	
	Hot pepper sauce, to taste (see Tip)	

1. In slow cooker stoneware, combine all ingredients except hot sauce. Stir thoroughly, cover and cook on Low for 8 hours or on High for 4 hours, until onions are tender.

2. Toss well with hot sauce and serve.

FOOD CHOICE VALUES PER SERVING

1/2 ◧ Fruit & Vegetable Choice

1/2 ▲ Fats & Oils Choice

NUTRIENT ANALYSIS PER SERVING

Calories	49	Fat, total	2 g
Carbohydrates	7 g	Fat, saturated	0 g
Fiber	1 g	Sodium	7 mg
Protein	1 g	Cholesterol	0 mg

New Orleans Braised Onions (page 128)
Overleaf: Moors and Christians (page 114)

Tips

Gnocchi is the Italian version of dumplings, usually made from potatoes or flour. This sweet potato version is served the traditional way with a sauce. It makes a wonderful side dish.

The sweet potatoes help to make this recipe an excellent source of vitamin A and E.

Sweet Potato Gnocchi with Parmesan Sauce

1½ lbs	sweet potatoes, scrubbed	750 g
⅓ cup	5% ricotta cheese	75 mL
1	large egg	1
¼ tsp	ground cinnamon	1 mL
⅛ tsp	freshly ground black pepper	0.5 mL
Pinch	salt	Pinch
1½ cups	all-purpose flour	375 mL

PARMESAN SAUCE

2 tsp	margarine or butter	10 mL
1½ tbsp	all-purpose flour	20 mL
1 cup	low-fat milk	250 mL
⅔ cup	vegetable stock (see recipe, page 28) or chicken stock	150 mL
3 tbsp	grated low-fat Parmesan cheese	45 mL

1. In a saucepan over medium-high heat, cover sweet potatoes with cold water; bring to a boil. Cook for 30 minutes or until tender when pierced with a fork; drain. When cool enough to handle, peel potatoes; mash. Add ricotta cheese, egg, cinnamon, pepper and salt; mash until well combined. Mix in flour.

2. On a lightly floured wooden board, roll about one-quarter of dough into a rope as thick as your thumb. With a sharp knife, cut into ¾-inch (2 cm) pieces. Repeat with remaining dough. Keep gnocchi pieces separate to avoid sticking.

3. In a large pot of boiling water, cook gnocchi (in batches of about 20) for 3 minutes or until they rise to the top; cook for another 30 seconds. Remove with a slotted spoon to a warm serving dish.

continued on page 131

FOOD CHOICE VALUES PER SERVING

2	■	Starch Choices
½	◆	Fruit & Vegetable Choice
½	◉	Protein Choice
½	▲	Fats & Oils Choice

NUTRIENT ANALYSIS PER SERVING			
Calories	214	Fat, total	4 g
Carbohydrates	39 g	Fat, saturated	1 g
Fiber	3 g	Sodium	115 mg
Protein	7 g	Cholesterol	33 mg

4. *Sauce:* In a small nonstick saucepan, heat margarine over low heat. Add flour; cook, stirring, for 1 minute. Add milk and stock; bring to a boil, whisking constantly. Reduce heat to low; cook for 5 minutes. Remove from heat. Add Parmesan cheese.

5. In a serving bowl combine gnocchi and sauce; toss well. Serve immediately.

New Potato Curry

2 tbsp	vegetable oil or clarified butter	25 mL
1 lb	small new potatoes, about 10 new potatoes (see Tip)	500 g
2	onions, finely chopped	2
1	clove garlic, minced	1
1 tsp	curry powder, preferably Madras	5 mL
1/2 tsp	salt	2 mL
1/2 tsp	cracked black peppercorns	2 mL
1/2 cup	water or vegetable or chicken stock	125 mL
2 tbsp	lemon juice	25 mL
1/4 cup	finely chopped cilantro	50 mL

1. In a skillet, heat butter or oil over medium-high heat. Add potatoes and cook just until they begin to brown. Transfer to slow cooker stoneware.

2. Reduce heat to medium. Add onions and cook, stirring, until softened. Add garlic, curry powder, salt and pepper. Stir and cook for 1 minute. Add water or stock, bring to a boil and pour over potatoes.

3. Cover and cook on Low for 8 to 10 hours or on High for 4 to 5 hours, until potatoes are tender. Stir in lemon juice and garnish with cilantro.

SERVES 6

Slow cooker

Tip
Leave the skins on potatoes, scrub thoroughly and dry on paper towels. Cut in half any that are larger than 1 inch (2.5 cm) in diameter.

Make ahead
This dish can be partially prepared the night before it is cooked. Complete Steps 1 and 2 and refrigerate overnight. The next day, continue cooking as directed in Step 3.

FOOD CHOICE VALUES PER SERVING

1 ■ Starch Choice

1 ▲ Fats & Oils Choice

NUTRIENT ANALYSIS PER SERVING			
Calories	111	Fat, total	4 g
Carbohydrates	17 g	Fat, saturated	3 g
Fiber	2 g	Sodium	288 mg
Protein	3 g	Cholesterol	10 mg

Originally from Russia, kasha is the name given to buckwheat seeds that have been hulled and, most often, either finely or coarsely ground. (Despite its name, buckwheat isn't a type of wheat; in fact, it is not a cereal at all.) Toasting the kernels enhances their nutty flavor and keeps them from sticking together.

This recipe is an excellent source of vitamin A and C, niacin and folic acid, as well as iron, magnesium and phosphorus.

Kasha with Beans and Salsa Dressing

DRESSING

½ cup	chopped fresh coriander	125 mL
⅓ cup	medium salsa	75 mL
¼ cup	low-fat sour cream	50 mL
3 tbsp	light mayonnaise	45 mL
2 tbsp	water	25 mL
1 tsp	minced garlic	5 mL

SALAD

1½ cups	vegetable stock (see recipe, page 28) or chicken stock	375 mL
¾ cup	whole grain kasha	175 mL
½ cup	canned red kidney beans, rinsed and drained	125 mL
½ cup	canned chickpeas, rinsed and drained	125 mL
½ cup	chopped red onions	125 mL

1. *Dressing:* In a bowl combine coriander, salsa, sour cream, mayonnaise, water and garlic. Set aside.

2. *Salad:* In a saucepan over high heat, bring stock to boil. Meanwhile, in a nonstick saucepan set over medium-high heat, toast kasha for 1 minute. Add hot stock; return to a boil, stirring. Reduce heat to medium-low; cook, covered, for 10 minutes or until kasha is tender and liquid is absorbed. Set aside to cool.

3. In a serving bowl, combine cooled kasha, red kidney beans, chickpeas and red onions. Pour dressing over; toss to coat well. Serve at room temperature or heat in microwave to serve warm.

FOOD CHOICE VALUES PER SERVING

2	■	Starch Choices
1	◢	Fruit & Vegetable Choice
½	◪	Protein Choice
½	▲	Fats & Oils Choice

NUTRIENT ANALYSIS PER SERVING			
Calories	238	Fat, total	5 g
Carbohydrates	42 g	Fat, saturated	0 g
Fiber	3 g	Sodium	210 mg
Protein	9 g	Cholesterol	0 mg

Just For Kids

Tips
Ground chicken,
turkey or veal can
replace the beef.

Chick peas can
be replaced with
kidney beans.

Make Ahead
Prepare up to a day
ahead, adding more
stock if too thick.
Great for leftovers.

Spicy Meatball and Pasta Stew

MEATBALLS

8 oz	lean ground beef	250 g
1	egg	1
2 tbsp	ketchup or chili sauce	25 mL
2 tbsp	seasoned bread crumbs	25 mL
1 tsp	minced garlic	5 mL
½ tsp	chili powder	2 mL

STEW

2 tsp	vegetable oil	10 mL
1 tsp	minced garlic	5 mL
1¼ cups	chopped onions	300 mL
¾ cup	chopped carrots	175 mL
3½ cups	low-sodium beef stock	875 mL
1	can (19 oz/540 mL) tomatoes, crushed	1
¾ cup	canned chick peas, drained	175 mL
1 tbsp	tomato paste	15 mL
2 tsp	granulated sugar	10 mL
2 tsp	chili powder	10 mL
1 tsp	dried oregano	5 mL
1¼ tsp	dried basil	6 mL
⅔ cup	small shell pasta	150 mL

1. *Meatballs:* In large bowl, combine ground beef, egg, ketchup, bread crumbs, garlic and chili powder; mix well. Form each ½ tbsp (7 mL) into a meatball and place on a baking sheet; cover and set aside.

continued on page 135

FOOD CHOICE VALUES PER SERVING

1 ■ Starch Choice

½ ◗ Fruit & Vegetable
   Choice

1 ◉ Protein Choice

1 ▲ Fats & Oils
   Choice

NUTRIENT ANALYSIS PER SERVING			
Calories	203	Fat, total	7 g
Carbohydrates	26 g	Fat, saturated	2 g
Fiber	3 g	Sodium	564 mg
Protein	11 g	Cholesterol	43 mg

2. *Stew:* In large nonstick saucepan, heat oil over medium heat. Add garlic, onions and carrots and cook for 5 minutes or until onions are softened. Stir in stock, tomatoes, chick peas, tomato paste, sugar, chili powder, oregano and basil; bring to a boil, reduce heat to medium-low, cover and let cook for 20 minutes. Bring to a boil again and stir in pasta and meatballs; let simmer for 10 minutes or until pasta is tender but firm, and meatballs are cooked.

Potato Wedge Fries

3	potatoes (about 10 oz/300 g each)	3
2 tbsp	melted margarine or butter	25 mL
1 tsp	minced garlic	5 mL
2 tbsp	grated Parmesan cheese	25 mL
1/4 tsp	paprika	1 mL

1. Scrub potatoes and cut lengthwise into 8 wedges. Put on prepared baking sheet. Combine margarine and garlic in a small bowl. Combine Parmesan and paprika in another small bowl.

2. Brush potato wedges with half of the margarine and cheese mixture. Bake for 20 minutes, turn the wedges, brush with remaining margarine mixture (reheat if necessary). Sprinkle on remaining Parmesan mixture, and bake for another 20 minutes or just until potatoes are tender and crisp.

SERVES 6

Preheat oven to 375°F (190°C)

Baking sheet sprayed with vegetable spray

Tip

If children like spicier fries, use chili powder instead of paprika.

Make Ahead

Cut potatoes early in the day and leave in cold water so they don't discolor.

FOOD CHOICE VALUES PER SERVING

1 ■ Starch Choice

1 ▲ Fats & Oils Choice

NUTRIENT ANALYSIS PER SERVING			
Calories	118	Fat, total	5 g
Carbohydrates	17 g	Fat, saturated	1 g
Fiber	1 g	Sodium	92 mg
Protein	3 g	Cholesterol	2 mg

Preheat oven to
350°F (180°C)

10- to 11-inch (25- to
28-cm) pizza or springform
baking pan sprayed
with vegetable spray

Make Ahead
Prepare pasta crust
and sauce early in day.
Do not pour sauce over
top until ready to bake.

Pizza Pasta with Beef-Tomato Sauce and Cheese

6 oz	macaroni	150 g
1	egg	1
1/3 cup	2% milk	75 mL
3 tbsp	grated Parmesan cheese	45 mL
1 tsp	vegetable oil	5 mL
2 tsp	crushed garlic	10 mL
3/4 cup	finely chopped onions	175 mL
1/2 cup	finely chopped sweet green peppers	125 mL
1/3 cup	finely chopped carrots	75 mL
8 oz	ground beef or chicken	250 g
1	can (19 oz/540 mL) tomatoes, crushed	1
2 tbsp	tomato paste	25 mL
1 1/2 tsp	dried basil	7 mL
1 tsp	dried oregano	5 mL
1 cup	low-fat mozzarella cheese, shredded	250 mL

1. Cook pasta in boiling water according to package instructions or until firm to the bite. Drain and place in serving bowl. Add egg, milk and cheese. Mix well. Place in baking pan as a crust and bake for 20 minutes.

2. Meanwhile, in medium nonstick saucepan sprayed with vegetable spray, heat oil; sauté garlic, onions, green peppers and carrots until tender, approximately 5 minutes. Add beef and sauté until no longer pink, approximately 4 minutes. Add tomatoes, paste, basil and oregano. Cover and simmer on low heat for 15 minutes, stirring occasionally.

3. Pour sauce into pasta crust. Sprinkle with cheese; bake for 10 minutes or until cheese melts.

FOOD CHOICE VALUES PER SERVING

1 ■ Starch Choice

1 ◢ Fruit & Vegetable Choice

2½ ◕ Protein Choices

1 ▲ Fats & Oils Choice

NUTRIENT ANALYSIS PER SERVING			
Calories	303	Fat, total	13 g
Carbohydrates	27 g	Fat, saturated	6 g
Fiber	2 g	Sodium	435 mg
Protein	20 g	Cholesterol	67 mg

Beef, Macaroni and Cheese Casserole

1 1/2 tsp	vegetable oil	7 mL
2 tsp	crushed garlic	10 mL
1/2 cup	chopped onion	125 mL
12 oz	lean ground beef	375 g
1	can (19 oz/540 mL) tomatoes, crushed	1
1 tsp	dried basil	5 mL
1 tsp	dried oregano	5 mL
1 cup	macaroni	250 mL
2 tbsp	grated Parmesan cheese	25 mL

1. In a large nonstick skillet, heat oil; sauté garlic and onion for 3 minutes. Add beef and sauté until no longer pink, stirring constantly to break up beef.

2. Add tomatoes, basil and oregano; cover and cook for 15 minutes, stirring occasionally.

3. Meanwhile, cook macaroni according to package directions or until firm to the bite. Drain and place in serving bowl. Toss with sauce and sprinkle with cheese.

FOOD CHOICE VALUES PER SERVING

1 1/2 ■ Starch Choice

1/2 ✦ Fruit & Vegetable Choice

2 1/2 ◉ Protein Choices

2 ▲ Fats & Oils Choices

NUTRIENT ANALYSIS PER SERVING			
Calories	359	Fat, total	16 g
Carbohydrates	32 g	Fat, saturated	6 g
Fiber	3 g	Sodium	436 mg
Protein	22 g	Cholesterol	50 mg

Beef-Stuffed Spuds

Tip

How to bake potatoes:
Scrub baking potatoes
(10 oz [300 g] each) well
and pierce skins with a
fork in several places to
allow steam to escape.
Place in 400°F (200°C)
oven for 1 hour or until
potatoes give slightly
when squeezed.

4	large potatoes (about 10 oz/300 g each)	4
8 oz	lean ground beef or ground veal	250 g
1/3 cup	finely chopped onions	75 mL
1	clove garlic, minced	1
1 tsp	Worcestershire sauce	5 mL
	Salt and pepper	
1/2 cup	sour cream or plain yogurt or buttermilk (approx.)	125 mL
2 tbsp	chopped parsley	25 mL
1 cup	shredded reduced-fat Cheddar cheese	250 mL

1. Bake potatoes as directed (see Tip).

2. In a large nonstick skillet over medium-high heat, cook beef, breaking up with back of spoon, for 4 minutes or until no longer pink.

3. Reduce heat to medium. Add onions, garlic and Worcestershire sauce; season with salt and pepper. Cook, stirring often, for 4 minutes or until onions are softened.

4. Cut warm potatoes into half lengthwise. Carefully scoop out each potato, leaving a 1/4-inch (5 mm) shell; set aside.

5. In a bowl mash potatoes with a potato masher or fork; beat in enough sour cream to make smooth. Stir in beef mixture, parsley and half the cheese; season to taste with salt and pepper. Spoon into potato shells; top with remaining cheese.

6. Arrange in baking dish; bake in preheated oven for 15 minutes or until cheese is melted. Alternatively, place on microwave-safe rack or large serving plate; microwave at Medium-High for 5 to 7 minutes or until heated through and cheese melts.

FOOD CHOICE VALUES PER SERVING

2 ■ Starch Choices

1 ⊘ Protein Choice

1/2 ▲ Fats & Oils Choice

NUTRIENT ANALYSIS PER SERVING			
Calories	227	Fat, total	6 g
Carbohydrates	31 g	Fat, saturated	3 g
Fiber	3 g	Sodium	101 mg
Protein	12 g	Cholesterol	22 mg

Preheat oven to
425°F (220°C)

Baking sheet sprayed
with vegetable spray

Tips

Children devour these
tasty egg rolls. Double
the recipe if necessary.

Ground chicken or veal
can replace beef.

Cheddar cheese can
replace mozzarella for a
more intense flavor.

Roll the wrappers
any way that's easy.
Wetting the edges of
the wrappers with water
may help secure roll.

Make Ahead

Prepare these up to
a day ahead and keep
refrigerated. Bake an
extra 5 minutes. These
can also be prepared and
frozen for up to a month.

FOOD CHOICE VALUES PER SERVING

2 ● Fruit & Vegetable Choices

1 ◕ Protein Choice

½ ▲ Fats & Oils Choice

1 ✦✦ Extra Choice

Italian Pizza Egg Rolls

1 tsp	vegetable oil	5 mL
1 tsp	minced garlic	5 mL
¼ cup	finely chopped carrots	50 mL
¼ cup	finely chopped onions	50 mL
¼ cup	finely chopped green peppers	50 mL
3 oz	lean ground beef	75 g
½ cup	tomato pasta sauce	125 mL
½ cup	grated mozzarella cheese (1 ½ oz/40g)	125 mL
1 tbsp	grated Parmesan cheese	15 mL
9	egg roll wrappers (5½ inches/13 cm square)	9

1. In nonstick skillet sprayed with vegetable spray, heat oil over medium heat. Add garlic, carrots and onions; cook for 8 minutes, or until softened and browned. Add peppers and cook 2 minutes longer. Add beef and cook for 2 minutes, stirring to break it up, or until it is no longer pink. Remove from heat and stir in tomato sauce, mozzarella and Parmesan cheeses.

2. Keeping rest of wrappers covered with a cloth to prevent drying out, put one wrapper on work surface with a corner pointing towards you. Put 2 tbsp (25 mL) of the filling in the center. Fold the lower corner up over the filling, fold the 2 side corners in over the filling, and roll the bundle away from you. Put on prepared pan and repeat until all wrappers are filled. Bake for 14 minutes, until browned, turning the pizza rolls at the halfway mark.

NUTRIENT ANALYSIS PER SERVING			
Calories	184	Fat, total	6 g
Carbohydrates	23 g	Fat, saturated	3 g
Fiber	1 g	Sodium	332 mg
Protein	10 g	Cholesterol	17 mg

Preheat oven to
400°F (200°C)

Baking sheet, with
greased rack

Tips

You can also make
extra batches of the
crumb mixture and
store in the freezer.

Instead of boneless
chicken breasts, prepare
skinless chicken
drumsticks in the same
way but bake in a 375°F
(190°C) oven for 35 to
40 minutes or until tender.

Adding salt brings the
sodium to 674 mg.

Yummy Parmesan Chicken Fingers

½ cup	finely crushed soda cracker crumbs (about 16 crackers)	125 mL
⅓ cup	freshly grated Parmesan cheese	75 mL
½ tsp	dried basil leaves	2 mL
½ tsp	dried marjoram leaves	2 mL
½ tsp	paprika	2 mL
½ tsp	salt, optional	2 mL
¼ tsp	freshly ground black pepper	1 mL
4	skinless, boneless chicken breasts	4
1	egg	1
2 tbsp	margarine or butter	25 mL
1	clove garlic, minced	1

1. In a food processor, combine cracker crumbs, Parmesan cheese, basil, marjoram, paprika, optional salt and pepper. Process to make fine crumbs. Place in a shallow bowl.

2. Cut chicken breasts into four strips each. In a bowl, beat egg; add chicken strips. Using a fork, dip chicken strips in crumb mixture until evenly coated. Arrange on greased rack set on baking sheet. In small bowl, microwave butter and garlic at High for 45 seconds or until melted. Brush chicken strips with melted butter.

3. Bake in preheated oven for 15 minutes or until no longer pink in center. (If frozen, bake for up to 25 minutes.)

FOOD CHOICE VALUES PER SERVING

½ ■ Starch Choice

3 ◉ Protein Choices

½ ▲ Fats & Oils Choice

NUTRIENT ANALYSIS PER SERVING

Calories	236	Fat, total	12 g
Carbohydrates	10 g	Fat, saturated	6 g
Fiber	1 g	Sodium	400 mg
Protein	22 g	Cholesterol	114 mg

Preheat oven to
400°F (200°C)

Foil-lined cookie
sheet, greased

Tips

Kids will love eating
these "fingers" with
their fingers.

This honey dip adds
about 20 g carbohydrate
or 2 ✳ Sugars Choices
to the meal. Choosing
another type of dip, such
as salsa, barbecue sauce
or low-fat dressing
can eliminate these
from the recipe.

Make Ahead

The chicken fingers and
honey dip can be made
up to 4 hours ahead,
covered and refrigerated.

Sesame Chicken Fingers with Honey Dip

HONEY DIP

1/3 cup	light mayonnaise	75 mL
3 tbsp	liquid honey	45 mL
1 tbsp	fresh lemon juice	15 mL
1/4 cup	light mayonnaise	50 mL
2 tbsp	Dijon mustard	25 mL
2 tbsp	fresh lemon juice	25 mL
1/3 cup	dry bread crumbs	75 mL
3 tbsp	sesame seeds	45 mL
1 tsp	dried Italian herb seasoning	5 mL
1 lb	skinless boneless chicken breasts, cut into strips 2 inches (5 cm) long by 1/2 inch (1 cm) wide	500 g

1. *Honey Dip:* In a bowl, stir together mayonnaise, honey and lemon juice until well combined. Refrigerate if making ahead.

2. In a bowl combine mayonnaise, Dijon mustard and lemon juice.

3. On waxed paper or in a bowl, combine bread crumbs, sesame seeds and Italian seasoning.

4. Coat chicken with mayonnaise mixture, then with bread crumb mixture. Place on prepared cookie sheet. Bake in preheated oven, turning once, for 15 to 20 minutes or until golden brown and chicken is no longer pink inside. Serve hot with the honey dip.

FOOD CHOICE VALUES PER SERVING

1/2 ▣ Starch Choice

2 ✳ Sugars Choices

4 ◪ Protein Choices

1/2 ▲ Fats & Oils Choice

NUTRIENT ANALYSIS PER SERVING			
Calories	367	Fat, total	15 g
Carbohydrates	31 g	Fat, saturated	2 g
Fiber	2 g	Sodium	422 mg
Protein	28 g	Cholesterol	66 mg

Turkey Macaroni Chili

Tips
Great mild-tasting
chili that children love.
Can be served as
a soup or alongside
rice or pasta.

Ground turkey can be
replaced with ground
chicken, beef or veal.

Red kidney beans can
be replaced with white
beans or chick peas.

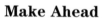

Make Ahead
Can be prepared up
to 2 days ahead and
reheated. Can be frozen
for up to 3 weeks.

Great for leftovers.

1 ½ tsp	vegetable oil	7 mL
1 tsp	minced garlic	5 mL
½ cup	finely chopped carrots	125 mL
1 cup	chopped onions	250 mL
8 oz	ground turkey	250 g
1	can (19 oz/540 mL) tomatoes, crushed	1
2 cups	chicken stock	500 mL
1 ½ cups	peeled, diced potatoes	375 mL
¾ cup	canned red kidney beans, drained	175 mL
¾ cup	corn kernels	175 mL
2 tbsp	tomato paste	25 mL
1 ½ tsp	chili powder	7 mL
1 ½ tsp	dried oregano	7 mL
1 ½ tsp	dried basil	7 mL
⅓ cup	elbow macaroni	75 mL

1. In large nonstick saucepan, heat oil over medium heat; add garlic, carrots and onions and cook for 8 minutes or until softened, stirring occasionally. Add turkey and cook, stirring to break it up, for 2 minutes or until no longer pink. Add tomatoes, stock, potatoes, beans, corn, tomato paste, chili, oregano and basil; bring to a boil, reduce heat to low, cover and simmer for 20 minutes.

2. Bring to a boil and add macaroni; cook for 12 minutes or until pasta is tender but firm.

FOOD CHOICE VALUES PER SERVING

1 ■ Starch Choice

1 ◧ Fruit & Vegetable Choice

1 ◧ Protein Choice

NUTRIENT ANALYSIS PER SERVING			
Calories	182	Fat, total	4 g
Carbohydrates	28 g	Fat, saturated	1 g
Fiber	4 g	Sodium	557 mg
Protein	10 g	Cholesterol	22 mg

Sweet and Sour Chicken Meatballs over Rice

Tips
If your kids don't like rice, serve this dish over 1 lb (500 g) spaghetti. Also, feel free to omit the onions.

Serve with 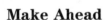 Extra vegetables such as green beans and add a ◆ Milk Choice to make this a complete meal.

Make Ahead
Make up to 2 days ahead; reheat before serving. Can be frozen for up to 6 weeks. Great for leftovers.

12 oz	ground chicken	375 g
1/4 cup	finely chopped onions	50 mL
2 tbsp	ketchup	25 mL
2 tbsp	bread crumbs	25 mL
1	egg	1
2 tsp	olive oil	10 mL
2 tsp	minced garlic	10 mL
1/3 cup	chopped onions	75 mL
2 cups	tomato juice	500 mL
2 cups	pineapple juice	500 mL
1/2 cup	chili sauce	125 mL
2 cups	white rice	500 mL

1. In a bowl combine chicken, onions, ketchup, bread crumbs and egg; mix well. Form each 1 tbsp (15 mL) mixture into a meatball; set aside.

2. In a large saucepan, heat oil over medium heat. Add garlic and onions; cook for 3 minutes or until softened. Add tomato juice, pineapple juice, chili sauce and meatballs. Simmer, covered, for 30 to 40 minutes or until meatballs are tender.

3. Meanwhile, bring 4 cups (1 L) water to boil; add rice. Reduce heat; simmer, covered, for 20 minutes or until liquid is absorbed. Remove from heat; let stand for 5 minutes, covered. Serve meatballs and sauce over rice.

FOOD CHOICE VALUES PER SERVING

2½ ■ Starch Choices

1½ ▨ Fruit & Vegetable Choices

1 ◢ Protein Choice

1 ▲ Fats & Oils Choice

NUTRIENT ANALYSIS PER SERVING			
Calories	346	Fat, total	8 g
Carbohydrates	54 g	Fat, saturated	1 g
Fiber	2 g	Sodium	422 mg
Protein	13 g	Cholesterol	27 mg

Preheat oven to
400°F (200°C)

Baking sheet sprayed
with vegetable spray

Tip

Use bran flakes instead
of natural bran; it has
a sweetness that
children love.

Make Ahead

Coat the drumsticks up
to 1 day ahead. They
can be baked a few hours
in advance and then
gently reheated. Great
for leftovers.

Crunchy Cheese and Herb Drumsticks

1½ cups	bran or corn flakes cereal	375 mL
1½ tbsp	fresh chopped parsley	20 mL
2½ tbsp	grated Parmesan cheese	35 mL
1 tsp	minced garlic	5 mL
¾ tsp	dried basil (or ½ tsp/2 mL dried)	4 mL
½ tsp	chili powder	2 mL
⅛ tsp	ground black pepper	0.5 mL
1	egg	1
2 tbsp	milk or water	25 mL
8	skinless chicken drumsticks	8

1. In a food processor combine bran flakes, parsley, Parmesan, garlic, basil, chili powder and pepper; process into fine crumbs. Set aside.

2. In a bowl whisk together egg and milk. Dip each drumstick into egg wash, then roll in crumbs; place on prepared baking sheet. Bake, turning halfway, for 35 minutes or until browned and chicken is cooked through.

FOOD CHOICE VALUES PER SERVING

½ ■ Starch Choice

4 ◙ Protein Choices

NUTRIENT ANALYSIS PER SERVING			
Calories	238	Fat, total	9 g
Carbohydrates	11 g	Fat, saturated	3 g
Fiber	2 g	Sodium	186 mg
Protein	28 g	Cholesterol	151 mg

Preheat oven to
375°F (190°C)

12 muffin cups sprayed
with vegetable spray

Tips
These muffins are
a heavenly treat for
children. What a
combination — peanut
butter, bananas
and chocolate!

Using 1/3 cup (75 mL)
granulated sugar and
1/3 cup (75 mL) sugar
substitute will change
the texture of the muffins
somewhat, but will
reduce the carbohydrate
content by 5 g per
serving and reduce the
✷ Sugars Choices to 1.

Make Ahead
Prepare up to a day
ahead. These freeze
well up to 4 weeks.

Banana Peanut Butter Chip Muffins

2/3 cup	granulated sugar	150 mL
3 tbsp	vegetable oil	45 mL
3 tbsp	peanut butter	45 mL
1	large banana, mashed	1
1	egg	1
1 tsp	vanilla	5 mL
3/4 cup	all-purpose flour	175 mL
3/4 tsp	baking powder	4 mL
3/4 tsp	baking soda	4 mL
1/4 cup	2% yogurt	50 mL
3 tbsp	semi-sweet chocolate chips	45 mL

1. In large bowl or food processor, combine sugar, oil, peanut butter, banana, egg and vanilla; mix until well blended. In another bowl combine flour, baking powder and baking soda; add to batter and mix just until blended. Stir in yogurt and chocolate chips.

2. Fill muffin cups half-full. Bake for 15 to 18 minutes, or until tops are firm to the touch and cake tester inserted in the center comes out dry.

FOOD CHOICE VALUES PER SERVING

1/2 ■ Starch Choice

1 1/2 ✷ Sugars Choices

2 ▲ Fats & Oils Choices

NUTRIENT ANALYSIS PER SERVING			
Calories	169	Fat, total	8 g
Carbohydrates	24 g	Fat, saturated	2 g
Fiber	1 g	Sodium	90 mg
Protein	3 g	Cholesterol	18 mg

Preheat oven to
350°F (180°C)

9-inch square (2.5 L)
pan sprayed with
vegetable spray

Tips
Chopped dates can
replace raisins.

Use a no sugar added
smooth or chunky
peanut butter.

Do not overcook the
peanut butter mixture.

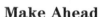

Make Ahead
Prepare these up to
2 days ahead and keep
tightly closed in a cookie
tin. These freeze for
up to 2 weeks.

Peanut Butter-Coconut-Raisin Granola Bars

1 ⅓ cups	rolled oats	325 mL
⅔ cup	raisins	150 mL
½ cup	bran flakes	125 mL
⅓ cup	unsweetened coconut	75 mL
3 tbsp	chocolate chips	45 mL
2 tbsp	chopped pecans	25 mL
1 tsp	baking soda	5 mL
¼ cup	peanut butter	50 mL
¼ cup	brown sugar	50 mL
3 tbsp	margarine or butter	45 mL
3 tbsp	honey	45 mL
1 tsp	vanilla	5 mL

1. Put oats, raisins, bran flakes, coconut, chocolate chips, pecans and baking soda in bowl. Combine until well mixed.

2. In small saucepan, whisk together peanut butter, brown sugar, margarine, honey and vanilla over medium heat for approximately 30 seconds or just until sugar dissolves and mixture is smooth. Pour over dry ingredients and stir to combine. Press into prepared pan and bake for 15 to 20 minutes or until browned. Let cool completely before cutting into bars.

FOOD CHOICE VALUES PER SERVING

½ ◆ Fruit & Vegetable Choice

½ ✳ Sugars Choice

1 ▲ Fats & Oils Choice

1 ✦✦ Extra Choice

NUTRIENT ANALYSIS PER SERVING			
Calories	97	Fat, total	5 g
Carbohydrates	13 g	Fat, saturated	2 g
Fiber	1 g	Sodium	77 mg
Protein	2 g	Cholesterol	0 mg

Breads, Biscuits, Muffins and More

Low-Fat Herbed Beer Bread

Tips

Fat-free and easy to
prepare, this loaf has a
delicate yeast flavor that
works well with soups,
salads and egg dishes.

Any type of beer
works well in this recipe
— whether cold or
at room temperature,
flat or foamy.

Variation

Increase the quantity
of one dried herb to
bring out the flavor
you like best.

2¾ cups	all-purpose flour	675 mL
2 tbsp	granulated sugar	25 mL
2 tbsp	baking powder	25 mL
1 tsp	salt	5 mL
½ tsp	dried marjoram	2 mL
½ tsp	dried oregano	2 mL
½ tsp	dried thyme	2 mL
Pinch	dried dill	Pinch
1	can (13 oz/355 mL) beer	1

1. In a large bowl, stir together flour, sugar, baking powder, salt, marjoram, oregano, thyme and dill. Add beer and stir just until combined. Spoon into prepared pan.

2. Bake in preheated oven for 70 to 80 minutes or until a cake tester inserted in the center comes out clean. Let cool in pan on rack for 10 minutes. Remove from pan and serve warm.

FOOD CHOICE VALUES PER SERVING (¹⁄₁₆ OF LOAF)

1 ▣ Starch Choice
½ ✳ Sugars Choice

NUTRIENT ANALYSIS PER SERVING

Calories	96	Fat, total	0 g
Carbohydrates	19 g	Fat, saturated	0 g
Fiber	1 g	Sodium	231 mg
Protein	2 g	Cholesterol	0 mg

Preheat oven to
400°F (200°C)

Baking sheet,
lightly greased

Tip

Score the top of the
round at least $\frac{1}{2}$ inch
(1 cm) deep. This will
ensure it breaks easily
into wedges.

Irish Whole Wheat Soda Bread

2 cups	whole wheat flour	500 mL
1 cup	all-purpose flour	250 mL
1 tbsp	granulated sugar	15 mL
1 tsp	baking powder	5 mL
1 tsp	baking soda	5 mL
1 tsp	salt	5 mL
1 $\frac{1}{2}$ cups	buttermilk	375 mL

1. In a large bowl, stir together whole wheat flour, flour, sugar, baking powder, baking soda and salt. Add buttermilk all at once, stirring with a fork to make a soft, but slightly sticky dough.

2. With lightly floured hands, form dough into a ball. On a lightly floured surface, knead the dough gently for 8 to 10 times. Pat the dough into a 6-inch (15 cm) thick round, with a slightly flattened top.

3. Place dough on prepared baking sheet. With a shape knife or pizza cutter, score the top in the shape of a cross or large X. Bake in preheated oven for 35 to 45 minutes. Remove from baking sheet onto a cooling rack immediately. Dust top with rice flour. Serve warm from the oven.

**FOOD CHOICE VALUES
PER SERVING
($\frac{1}{12}$ OF LOAF)**

$1\frac{1}{2}$ ■ Starch Choices

NUTRIENT ANALYSIS PER SERVING			
Calories	123	Fat, total	1 g
Carbohydrates	25 g	Fat, saturated	0 g
Fiber	3 g	Sodium	335 mg
Protein	5 g	Cholesterol	1 mg

Preheat oven to
350°F (180°C)

9- by 5-inch (2 L)
loaf pan, lightly greased

Tip

Leave blueberries in the
freezer until just before
using. This will help to
prevent them from
"bleeding" into the bread.

Variation

Try substituting half or
all of the blueberries with
frozen sour cherries
or cranberries.

Blueberry Buckwheat Bread

1²⁄₃ cups	all-purpose flour	400 mL
¹⁄₃ cup	buckwheat flour	75 mL
1 tbsp	baking powder	15 mL
¹⁄₂ tsp	salt	2 mL
1 tsp	grated lemon zest	5 mL
3 tbsp	vegetable oil	45 mL
2	egg whites	2
1¹⁄₄ cups	plain yogurt	300 mL
¹⁄₃ cup	honey	75 mL
¹⁄₂ cup	frozen blueberries	125 mL

1. In a large bowl, stir together flour, buckwheat flour, baking powder, salt and zest.

2. In a separate bowl, using an electric mixer, beat oil, eggs, yogurt and honey until combined. Pour mixture over dry ingredients and stir just until combined. Gently fold in frozen blueberries. Spoon into prepared pan.

3. Bake in preheated oven for 70 to 80 minutes or until a cake tester inserted in the center comes out clean. Let cool in pan on rack for 10 minutes. Remove from pan and let cool completely on rack.

FOOD CHOICE VALUES PER SERVING (¹⁄₁₂ OF LOAF)

1	■	Starch Choice
1	✳	Sugars Choice
¹⁄₂	▲	Fats & Oils Choice
1	✦✦	Extra Choice

NUTRIENT ANALYSIS PER SERVING

Calories	158	Fat, total	4 g
Carbohydrates	28 g	Fat, saturated	0 g
Fiber	1 g	Sodium	181 mg
Protein	4 g	Cholesterol	0 mg

Fruited Barm Brack

2 cups	all-purpose flour	500 mL
½ cup	packed brown sugar	125 mL
2 tsp	baking powder	10 mL
½ tsp	baking soda	2 mL
½ tsp	salt	2 mL
1 tsp	ground cinnamon	5 mL
1 tsp	ground nutmeg	5 mL
½ cup	snipped dried apricots	125 mL
½ cup	currants	125 mL
½ cup	dried cranberries	125 mL
2 tbsp	vegetable oil	25 mL
1	egg	1
1 cup	tea (at room temperature)	250 mL

1. In a large bowl, stir together flour, brown sugar, baking powder, baking soda, salt, cinnamon and nutmeg. Stir in dried apricots, currants and dried cranberries.

2. In a separate bowl, using an electric mixer, beat oil, egg and tea until combined. Pour mixture over dry ingredients and stir just until combined. Spoon into prepared pan.

3. Bake in preheated oven for 70 to 80 minutes or until a cake tester inserted in the center comes out clean. Let cool in pan on rack for 10 minutes. Remove from pan and let cool completely on rack.

NUTRIENT ANALYSIS PER SERVING			
Calories	186	Fat, total	3 g
Carbohydrates	37 g	Fat, saturated	0 g
Fiber	2 g	Sodium	192 mg
Protein	3 g	Cholesterol	18 mg

Low-Fat Applesauce Raisin Bread

2 cups	all-purpose flour	500 mL
½ cup	granulated sugar	125 mL
1 tsp	baking powder	5 mL
½ tsp	baking soda	2 mL
¼ tsp	salt	1 mL
½ tsp	ground cinnamon	2 mL
1 cup	raisins	250 mL
2	egg whites	2
1¼ cups	unsweetened applesauce	300 mL

1. In a large bowl, stir together flour, sugar, baking powder, baking soda, salt and cinnamon. Stir in raisins.

2. In a separate bowl, using an electric mixer, beat egg whites and applesauce until combined. Pour mixture over dry ingredients and stir just until combined. Spoon into prepared pan.

3. Bake in preheated oven for 70 to 80 minutes or until a cake tester inserted in the center comes out clean. Let cool in pan on rack for 10 minutes. Remove from pan and let cool completely on rack.

**FOOD CHOICE VALUES
PER SERVING
(¹⁄₁₆ OF LOAF)**

1 ■ Starch Choice

1 ✔ Fruit & Vegetable
Choice

NUTRIENT ANALYSIS PER SERVING

Calories	123	Fat, total	0 g
Carbohydrates	29 g	Fat, saturated	0 g
Fiber	1 g	Sodium	95 mg
Protein	2 g	Cholesterol	0 mg

Preheat oven to
350°F (180°C)

9- by 5-inch (2 L)
loaf pan, lightly greased

Variation
Substitute sesame
or flaxseeds for the
poppy seeds.

Poppy Seed Oat Bread

1 cup	whole wheat flour	250 mL
1 cup	all-purpose flour	250 mL
1 cup	quick-cooking oats	250 mL
1 tsp	baking powder	5 mL
1 tsp	baking soda	5 mL
1/2 tsp	salt	2 mL
1/4 cup	poppy seeds	50 mL
1	egg	1
1 3/4 cups	buttermilk	425 mL
1/3 cup	honey	75 mL

1. In a large bowl, stir together whole wheat flour, flour, oats, baking powder, baking soda, salt and poppy seeds.

2. In a separate bowl, using an electric mixer, beat egg and buttermilk until combined. Add honey while mixing. Pour mixture over dry ingredients and stir just until combined. Spoon into prepared pan.

3. Bake in preheated oven for 70 to 80 minutes or until a cake tester inserted in the center comes out clean. Let cool in pan on rack for 10 minutes. Remove from pan and let cool completely on rack.

**FOOD CHOICE VALUES
PER SERVING
(1/12 OF LOAF)**

1 1/2 ■ Starch Choices

1 ✳ Sugars Choice

1/2 ◪ Protein Choice

NUTRIENT ANALYSIS PER SERVING			
Calories	174	Fat, total	3 g
Carbohydrates	32 g	Fat, saturated	1 g
Fiber	2 g	Sodium	254 mg
Protein	6 g	Cholesterol	19 mg

Preheat oven to
350°F (180°C)

9- by 5-inch (2 L)
loaf pan, lightly greased

Tip

Leave blueberries in
the freezer until just
before using. This will
help to prevent them
from "bleeding" into the
bread. Use ripe bananas
for the best flavor.

Variation

Try natural wheat bran
instead of the oat bran.

Blueberry Banana Oat Bread

1¾ cups	all-purpose flour	425 mL
¼ cup	quick-cooking oats	50 mL
2 tbsp	oat bran	25 mL
½ cup	granulated sugar	125 mL
2 tsp	baking powder	10 mL
½ tsp	salt	2 mL
2 tbsp	vegetable oil	25 mL
1	egg	1
1½ cups	mashed bananas	375 mL
¾ cup	frozen blueberries (see Tip)	175 mL

1. In a large bowl, stir together flour, oats, oat bran, sugar, baking powder and salt.

2. In a separate bowl, using an electric mixer, beat oil, egg and banana until combined. Pour mixture over dry ingredients and stir just until combined. Gently fold in frozen blueberries. Spoon into prepared pan.

3. Bake in preheated oven for 70 to 80 minutes or until a cake tester inserted in the center comes out clean. Let cool in pan on rack for 10 minutes. Remove from pan and serve warm.

**FOOD CHOICE VALUES
PER SERVING
(¹⁄₁₂ OF LOAF)**

1	■ Starch Choice
½	◗ Fruit & Vegetable Choice
1	✱ Sugars Choice
½	▲ Fats & Oils Choice

NUTRIENT ANALYSIS PER SERVING

Calories	169	Fat, total	3 g
Carbohydrates	32 g	Fat, saturated	0 g
Fiber	2 g	Sodium	138 mg
Protein	3 g	Cholesterol	18 mg

Preheat oven to
350°F (180°C)

9- by 5-inch (2 L)
loaf pan, lightly greased

Tip
The rhubarb must
be finely chopped;
otherwise, the finished
loaf tends to crumble
when sliced.

Variation
Substitute pecans
or pistachios for the
walnuts and lemon
zest for the orange.

Rhubarb Orange Bread

1¾ cups	finely chopped rhubarb	425 mL
⅓ cup	granulated sugar	75 mL
2 cups	all-purpose flour	500 mL
2 tsp	baking powder	10 mL
¾ tsp	baking soda	4 mL
½ tsp	salt	2 mL
2 tbsp	grated orange zest	25 mL
½ cup	chopped walnuts	125 mL
3 tbsp	vegetable oil	45 mL
1	egg	1
⅔ cup	orange juice	150 mL
1 tsp	vanilla extract	5 mL

1. In a bowl combine rhubarb and sugar; set aside for 10 to 15 minutes.

2. In a large bowl, stir together flour, baking powder, baking soda, salt and zest. Stir in walnuts.

3. In a separate bowl, using an electric mixer, beat oil, egg, juice and vanilla extract until combined. Stir in reserved rhubarb mixture. Pour over dry ingredients and stir just until combined. Spoon into prepared pan.

4. Bake in preheated oven for 70 to 80 minutes or until a cake tester inserted in the center comes out clean. Let cool in pan on rack for 10 minutes. Remove from pan and let cool completely on rack.

FOOD CHOICE VALUES PER SERVING (¹⁄₁₂ OF LOAF)

1½ ■ Starch Choices

1½ ▲ Fats & Oils Choices

1 ◆◆ Extra Choice

NUTRIENT ANALYSIS PER SERVING			
Calories	178	Fat, total	7 g
Carbohydrates	25 g	Fat, saturated	1 g
Fiber	1 g	Sodium	214 mg
Protein	4 g	Cholesterol	18 mg

Preheat oven to
350°F (180°C)

9- by 5-inch (2 L)
loaf pan, lightly greased

Tip
Blueberries are
becoming very popular as
a source of antioxidants
with disease-fighting
properties.

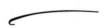

Variation
For a milder spice flavor,
use mace or nutmeg
instead of the cardamom.

Peach Blueberry Quick Bread

1¾ cups	all-purpose flour	425 mL
2½ tsp	baking powder	12 mL
¾ tsp	salt	4 mL
½ tsp	ground cardamom	2 mL
⅓ cup	margarine	75 mL
⅔ cup	granulated sugar	150 mL
2	eggs	2
⅓ cup	milk	75 mL
1 cup	chopped fresh peaches	250 mL
½ cup	fresh or frozen blueberries	125 mL

1. In a large bowl, stir together flour, baking powder, salt and cardamom.

2. In a separate large bowl, using an electric mixer, cream margarine, sugar and eggs until light and fluffy. Stir in dry ingredients alternately with milk, making 3 additions of dry ingredients and 2 of milk; stir just until combined. Gently fold in peaches and blueberries. Spoon into prepared pan.

3. Bake in preheated oven for 70 to 80 minutes or until a cake tester inserted in the center comes out clean. Let cool in pan on rack for 10 minutes. Remove from pan and let cool completely on rack.

**FOOD CHOICE VALUES
PER SERVING
(¹⁄₁₂ OF LOAF)**

1 ◼ Starch Choice

1 ✴ Sugars Choice

1 ▲ Fats & Oils Choice

1 ✚✚ Extra Choice

NUTRIENT ANALYSIS PER SERVING

Calories	180	Fat, total	6 g
Carbohydrates	28 g	Fat, saturated	1 g
Fiber	1 g	Sodium	266 mg
Protein	3 g	Cholesterol	36 mg

Russian Blini

$\frac{1}{3}$ cup	milk	75 mL
$\frac{1}{2}$ tsp	granulated sugar	2 mL
$\frac{1}{2}$ tsp	instant yeast	2 mL
1	egg yolk	1
1 tsp	vegetable oil	5 mL
$\frac{1}{3}$ cup	all-purpose flour	75 mL
2 tbsp	buckwheat flour	25 mL
$\frac{1}{4}$ tsp	salt	1 mL
2	egg whites	2
Pinch	cream of tartar	Pinch

1. In a small microwaveable bowl, heat milk to lukewarm. Stir in sugar and yeast.

2. In another bowl, whisk together egg yolk and oil. Add yeast mixture, flour, buckwheat flour and salt stirring until smooth. Cover and set in a pan of warm water for $1\frac{1}{4}$ hours.

3. In a separate bowl, using an electric mixer, beat egg whites and cream of tartar until stiff (but not dry) peaks form; using a spatula, fold whites gently into batter.

4. Heat pan until medium hot. Using 2 tbsp (25 mL) batter, spoon into hot pan. Spread batter, with the back of a spoon, for thinner blini. When the underside is brown, turn and cook about 30 to 60 seconds longer or until the second side is golden brown. Repeat with remaining batter.

NUTRIENT ANALYSIS PER SERVING			
Calories	42	Fat, total	1 g
Carbohydrates	6 g	Fat, saturated	0 g
Fiber	0 g	Sodium	78 mg
Protein	2 g	Cholesterol	24 mg

Scottish Oatmeal Scones

Preheat oven to
425°F (220°C)

Baking sheet,
lightly greased

1 cup	whole wheat flour	250 mL
1¼ cups	all-purpose flour	300 mL
½ cup	quick-cooking oats	125 mL
2 tsp	baking powder	10 mL
¾ tsp	salt	4 mL
⅓ cup	margarine	75 mL
1	egg	1
¾ cup	buttermilk	175 mL

Tip

To enjoy the next day,
split scones in half and
reheat in a toaster oven.

Variation

For a heavier, more
traditional oatmeal
biscuit, omit the
margarine. this
will eliminate the
 Fats & Oils Choice.

1. In a large bowl, stir together whole wheat flour, flour, oats, baking powder and salt. Using a pastry blender, cut in margarine until mixture resembles coarse crumbs.

2. In a small bowl, whisk together egg and buttermilk. Pour over dry ingredients all at once, stirring with a fork to make a soft, but slightly sticky dough.

3. With lightly floured hands, form dough into a ball. On a lightly floured surface, knead the dough gently for 8 to 10 times. Pat or roll out the dough into a 1-inch (2.5 cm) thick round.

4. Using a 2-inch (5 cm) floured biscuit cutter, cut out as many rounds as possible. Place on baking sheet. Gently form scraps into a ball, flatten and cut out rounds.

5. Bake in preheated oven for 12 to 15 minutes. Remove from baking sheet onto a cooling rack immediately. Serve warm.

FOOD CHOICE VALUES PER SERVING

1 ■ Starch Choice

1 ▲ Fats & Oils Choice

NUTRIENT ANALYSIS PER SERVING

Calories	133	Fat, total	5 g
Carbohydrates	18 g	Fat, saturated	1 g
Fiber	2 g	Sodium	225 mg
Protein	4 g	Cholesterol	16 mg

Preheat oven to
425°F (220°C)

Baking sheet,
lightly greased

Tip
Adjust the quantity of
poppy seeds to your
taste. For browner,
crisper tops, bake
biscuits in the upper
third of the oven.

Variation
Poppy seeds can
be replaced with any
other small seed – such
as sesame, caraway,
fennel, anise or mini
sunflower seeds. For
stronger-flavored seeds,
you may wish to reduce
the quantity used.

Whole Wheat Poppy Biscuits

1 ½ cups	whole wheat flour	375 mL
1 cup	all-purpose flour	250 mL
¼ cup	granulated sugar	50 mL
¼ cup	poppy seeds	50 mL
1 tbsp	baking powder	15 mL
½ tsp	baking soda	2 mL
½ tsp	salt	2 mL
⅓ cup	margarine	75 mL
1 cup	buttermilk	250 mL

1. In a large bowl, stir together whole wheat flour, flour, sugar, poppy seeds, baking powder, baking soda and salt. Using a pastry blender, cut in margarine until mixture resembles coarse crumbs. Add buttermilk all at once, stirring with a fork to make a soft, but slightly sticky dough.

2. With lightly floured hands, form dough into a ball. On a lightly floured surface, knead the dough gently for 8 to 10 times. Pat or roll out the dough into a ½-inch (1 cm) thick round.

3. Using a 2-inch (5 cm) floured biscuit cutter, cut out as many rounds as possible. Place on baking sheet. Gently form scraps into a ball, flatten and cut out rounds.

4. Bake in preheated oven for 12 to 15 minutes. Remove from baking sheet onto a cooling rack immediately. Serve warm.

FOOD CHOICE VALUES PER SERVING (1 BISCUIT)

1 ■ Starch Choice

1 ▲ Fats & Oils Choice

NUTRIENT ANALYSIS PER SERVING			
Calories	117	Fat, total	5 g
Carbohydrates	17 g	Fat, saturated	1 g
Fiber	2 g	Sodium	193 mg
Protein	3 g	Cholesterol	0 mg

Lemon Yogurt Biscuits

2 cups	all-purpose flour	500 mL
2 tbsp	granulated sugar	25 mL
1 tbsp	baking powder	15 mL
1/2 tsp	baking soda	2 mL
1/2 tsp	salt	2 mL
2 tsp	grated lemon zest	10 mL
1/3 cup	cold margarine or butter	75 mL
1 cup	plain yogurt	250 mL

1. In a large bowl, stir together flour, sugar, baking powder, baking soda, salt and zest. Using a pastry blender, cut in margarine until mixture resembles coarse crumbs. Add yogurt all at once, stirring with a fork to make a soft, but slightly sticky dough.

2. With lightly floured hands, form dough into a ball. On a lightly floured surface, knead the dough gently for 8 to 10 times. Pat or roll out the dough into a 1-inch (2.5 cm) thick round. Using a 2-inch (5 cm) floured cutter, cut out as many rounds as possible. Place on baking sheet. Gently form scraps into a ball, flatten and cut out rounds.

3. Bake in preheated oven for 12 to 15 minutes. Remove from baking sheet onto a cooling rack immediately.

FOOD CHOICE VALUES PER SERVING (1 BISCUIT)

1 ■ Starch Choice
1/2 ✳ Sugars Choice
1 ▲ Fats & Oils Choice

NUTRIENT ANALYSIS PER SERVING

Calories	141	Fat, total	5 g
Carbohydrates	20 g	Fat, saturated	1 g
Fiber	1 g	Sodium	281 mg
Protein	3 g	Cholesterol	0 mg

New Potato Curry (page 131)

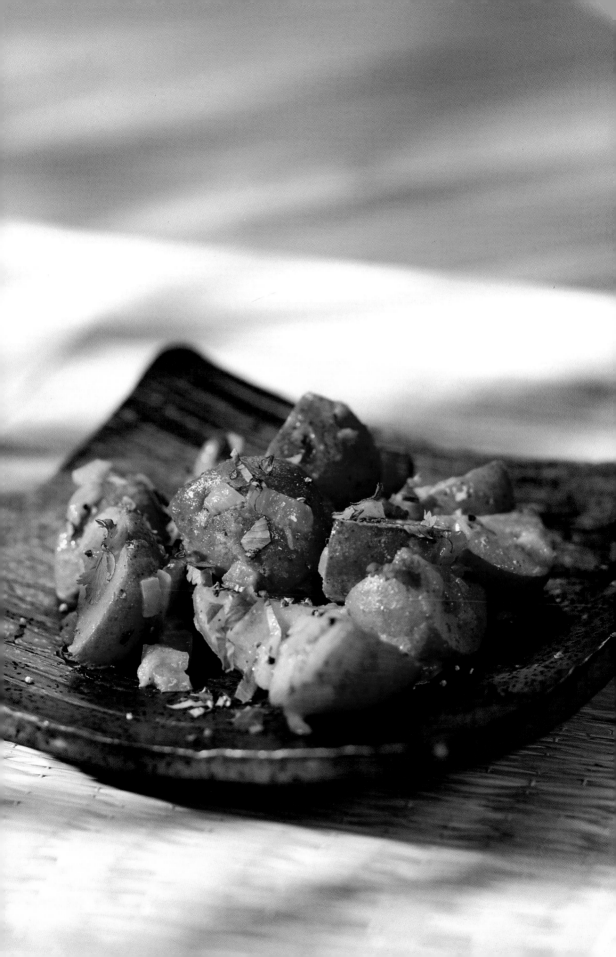

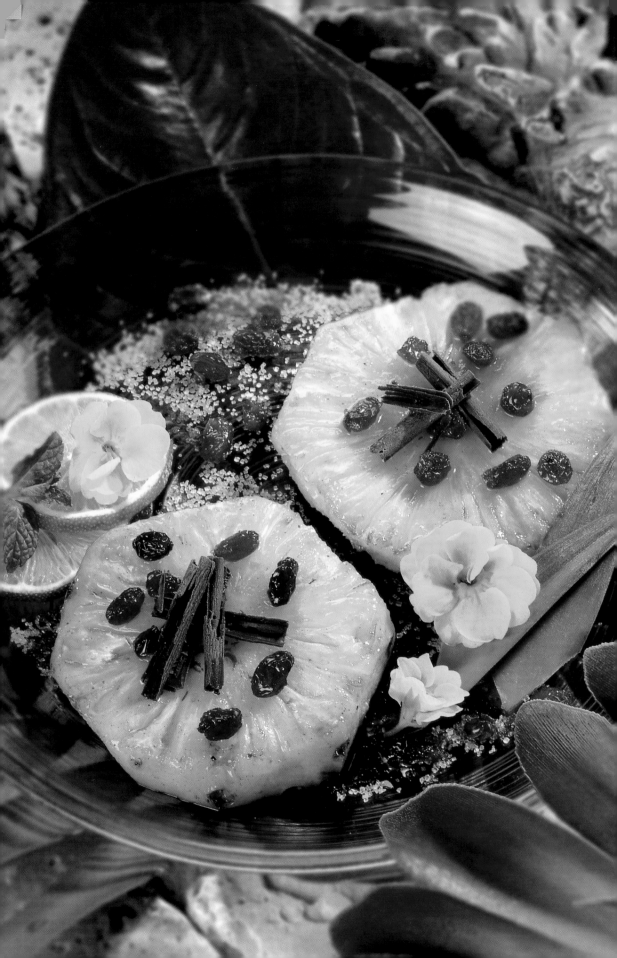

Wheat Muffins

Preheat oven to
400°F (200°C)

12-cup muffin tin, sprayed
with low-fat cooking
spray or paper-lined

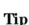

Tip
To keep muffins at their
best, freeze any which
won't be used in the first
2 days after baking. Thaw
at room temperature or
reheat in the microwave.

1 cup	all-purpose flour	250 mL
1 cup	unsifted whole-wheat flour	250 mL
2 tsp	baking powder	10 mL
1 tsp	salt	5 mL
1	egg, slightly beaten	1
¼ cup	molasses	50 mL
1 cup	milk	250 mL
¼ cup	margarine or butter, melted	50 mL

1. In a large bowl, combine all-purpose flour, whole-wheat flour, baking powder and salt. Make a well in the center.

2. In another bowl, combine egg, molasses, milk and margarine. Add to flour mixture, stirring just until blended. Do not overmix.

3. Spoon batter into prepared muffin tin, filling cups three-quarters full. Bake in preheated oven for 25 minutes or until golden brown.

**FOOD CHOICE VALUES
PER SERVING
(1 MUFFIN)**

1 ■ Starch Choice

½ ✳ Sugars Choice

1 ▲ Fats & Oils
Choice

NUTRIENT ANALYSIS PER SERVING			
Calories	138	Fat, total	5 g
Carbohydrates	21 g	Fat, saturated	1 g
Fiber	2 g	Sodium	290 mg
Protein	4 g	Cholesterol	18 mg

Fried Pineapple (page 180)

Preheat oven to
400°F (200°C)

12-cup muffin tin, sprayed
with low-fat cooking
spray or paper-lined

Honey Whole Wheat Muffins

1 cup	whole wheat flour	250 mL
1 cup	all-purpose flour	250 mL
3 tsp	baking powder	15 mL
1 tsp	salt	5 mL
1	egg	1
1 cup	milk	250 mL
¼ cup	vegetable oil	50 mL
¼ cup	honey	50 mL

1. In a large bowl, combine whole-wheat flour, all-purpose flour, baking powder and salt. Make a well in the center.

2. In another bowl, whisk together egg, milk and oil. Add the honey. Stir into flour mixture until moist and lumpy.

3. Spoon batter into prepared muffin tin, dividing evenly. Bake in preheated oven for 20 to 25 minutes or until lightly browned.

FOOD CHOICE VALUES PER SERVING (1 MUFFIN)

1 ■ Starch Choice

½ ✳ Sugars Choice

1 ▲ Fats & Oils Choice

NUTRIENT ANALYSIS PER SERVING

Calories	152	Fat, total	5 g
Carbohydrates	23 g	Fat, saturated	1 g
Fiber	2 g	Sodium	260 mg
Protein	4 g	Cholesterol	18 mg

Preheat oven to
400°F (200°C)

12-cup muffin tin, sprayed
with low-fat cooking
spray or paper-lined

Blueberry Wheat Germ Muffins

1¾ cups	all-purpose flour	425 mL
⅓ cup	wheat germ	75 mL
⅓ cup	granulated sugar	75 mL
1 tbsp	baking powder	15 mL
1½ tsp	grated lemon zest	7 mL
½ tsp	salt	2 mL
1	egg	1
1 cup	milk	250 mL
¼ cup	vegetable oil	50 mL
1 cup	fresh blueberries or frozen blueberries, drained	250 mL

1. In a large bowl, combine flour, wheat germ, sugar, baking powder, zest and salt. Make a well in the center.

2. In another bowl, whisk together egg, milk and oil. Add to dry ingredients, stirring just until moist and blended. Fold in berries.

3. Spoon batter into prepared muffin tin, filling cups three-quarters full. Bake in preheated oven for 20 to 25 minutes.

**FOOD CHOICE VALUES
PER SERVING
(1 MUFFIN)**

1 ■ Starch Choice

½ ◢ Fruit & Vegetable Choice

½ ✳ Sugars Choice

1 ▲ Fats & Oils Choice

NUTRIENT ANALYSIS PER SERVING			
Calories	161	Fat, total	6 g
Carbohydrates	24 g	Fat, saturated	1 g
Fiber	1 g	Sodium	170 mg
Protein	4 g	Cholesterol	18 mg

Preheat oven to
400°F (200°C)

12-cup muffin tin, sprayed
with low-fat cooking
spray or paper-lined

Peanut Butter Surprise Muffins

1 cup	all-purpose flour	250 mL
1/2 tsp	salt	2 mL
3 tsp	baking powder	15 mL
1 tbsp	granulated sugar	15 mL
1/2 cup	cornmeal	125 mL
1 cup	milk	250 mL
1	egg, beaten	1
1/4 cup	peanut butter	50 mL
1 tbsp	margarine or butter, melted	15 mL

1. In a large bowl, combine flour, salt, baking powder and sugar. Stir in cornmeal, mixing to blend well.

2. In a small bowl, combine milk, egg, peanut butter and melted margarine. Add to dry ingredients, stirring until moistened and blended.

3. Spoon batter into prepared muffin tin, filling cups three-quarters full. Bake in preheated oven for about 20 minutes.

FOOD CHOICE VALUES PER SERVING (1 MUFFIN)

1 ■ Starch Choice

1 ▲ Fats & Oils Choice

NUTRIENT ANALYSIS PER SERVING			
Calories	120	Fat, total	5 g
Carbohydrates	16 g	Fat, saturated	1 g
Fiber	1 g	Sodium	170 mg
Protein	4 g	Cholesterol	18 mg

Kiwi Raspberry Muffins

Preheat oven to
400°F (200°C)

12-cup muffin tin, sprayed
with low-fat cooking
spray or paper-lined

1 cup	all-purpose flour	250 mL
1 cup	whole-wheat flour	250 mL
1 tbsp	baking powder	15 mL
½ tsp	baking soda	2 mL
2	peeled chopped kiwi	2
½ cup	fresh raspberries (or frozen)	125 mL
1	egg, lightly beaten	1
¼ cup	margarine or butter	50 mL
⅓ cup	skim milk	75 mL
1 tsp	vanilla	5 mL

1. In a large bowl, mix together all-purpose flour, whole-wheat flour, baking powder and baking soda. Add kiwi and raspberries, mixing well. Make a well in the center.

2. In another bowl, combine egg, margarine, milk and vanilla. Add to the flour mixture, stirring only until moistened and blended. Do not overmix.

3. Spoon batter into prepared muffin tin, filling cups to the top. Bake in preheated oven for 15 to 20 minutes.

**FOOD CHOICE VALUES
PER SERVING
(1 MUFFIN)**

1 ■ Starch Choice

1 ▲ Fats & Oils
Choice

NUTRIENT ANALYSIS PER SERVING			
Calories	126	Fat, total	5 g
Carbohydrates	19 g	Fat, saturated	1 g
Fiber	2 g	Sodium	219 mg
Protein	3 g	Cholesterol	18 mg

Preheat oven to
350°F (180°C)

9-inch (2.5 L) springform
pan, lightly greased

Tip

Be sure to buy pumpkin
purée – not pumpkin pie
filling, which is too
sweet and contains
too much moisture for
this snacking cake.

Variation

Substitute 2 to
3 tsp (10 to 15 mL)
pumpkin pie spice for
the individual spices.

Orange Pumpkin Snacking Cake

1 cup	whole wheat flour	250 mL
2 cups	all-purpose flour	500 mL
¾ cup	packed brown sugar	175 mL
1 tbsp	grated orange zest	15 mL
1 tbsp	baking powder	15 mL
1 tsp	baking soda	5 mL
1 tsp	ground cinnamon	5 mL
½ tsp	ground allspice	2 mL
½ tsp	ground ginger	2 mL
½ tsp	ground nutmeg	2 mL
¼ tsp	ground cloves	1 mL
½ cup	vegetable oil	125 mL
3	eggs	3
1¼ cups	canned pumpkin purée (not pie filling)	300 mL
½ cup	orange juice	125 mL
1 cup	chopped pecans	250 mL

1. In a large bowl, stir together whole wheat flour, flour, brown sugar, zest, baking powder, baking soda, cinnamon, allspice, ginger, nutmeg and cloves; set aside.

2. In a separate bowl, using an electric mixer, beat oil, eggs, pumpkin purée and orange juice until combined. Pour mixture over dry ingredients and stir just until combined. Stir in pecans. Spoon into prepared pan.

3. Bake in preheated oven for 60 to 70 minutes or until a cake tester inserted in the center comes out clean. Immediately invert on a cooling rack. Remove pan and let cool completely.

**FOOD CHOICE VALUES
PER SERVING
(¹⁄₁₆ OF CAKE)**

1 ▪ Starch Choice

½ ▰ Fruit & Vegetable Choice

1 ✳ Sugars Choice

2½ ▲ Fats & Oils Choices

NUTRIENT ANALYSIS PER SERVING			
Calories	253	Fat, total	13 g
Carbohydrates	32 g	Fat, saturated	1 g
Fiber	2 g	Sodium	139 mg
Protein	5 g	Cholesterol	40 mg

Cookies and Desserts

Oat Bran Raisin Cookies

Preheat oven to
350°F (180°C)

Greased cookie sheet

Tip
This recipe makes a
smaller batch of cookies
than usual but it can be
doubled, if desired.

⅔ cup	uncooked oat bran cereal	160 mL
¼ cup	old-fashioned rolled oats	50 mL
3 tbsp	all-purpose flour	45 mL
½ tsp	baking powder	2 mL
3 tbsp	softened margarine	45 mL
¼ cup	firmly packed brown sugar	50 mL
1	egg white, lightly beaten	1
2 tsp	water	10 mL
¼ tsp	vanilla	1 mL
2 tbsp	raisins	25 mL

1. In a bowl, mix together oat bran, rolled oats, flour and baking powder.

2. In another bowl, beat together margarine and brown sugar until smooth and creamy. Stir in egg white, water and vanilla, mixing until thoroughly incorporated. Add flour mixture and mix well. Fold in raisins.

3. Drop by level tablespoonfuls (15 mL), about 2 inches (5 cm) apart, onto prepared cookie sheet. Using a fork or the bottom of a glass flatten slightly. Bake in preheated oven for 12 to 15 minutes or until bottoms are slightly browned. Cool on sheet for 3 minutes, then transfer to wire racks to cool completely.

**FOOD CHOICE VALUES
PER SERVING
(1 COOKIE)**

½ ■ Starch Choice

½ ✳ Sugars Choice

½ ▲ Fats & Oils Choice

NUTRIENT ANALYSIS PER SERVING			
Calories	86	Fat, total	4 g
Carbohydrates	12 g	Fat, saturated	1 g
Fiber	1 g	Sodium	53 mg
Protein	2 g	Cholesterol	0 mg

Preheat oven to
375°F (190°C)

Greased cookie sheet

Tip

Freeze cranberries
before chopping or
grinding them to
ease clean up.

Cranberry Orange Oatmeal Cookies

2 cups	all-purpose flour	500 mL
1 tsp	baking powder	5 mL
1/4 tsp	baking soda	1 mL
1/2 tsp	salt	2 mL
2 cups	quick-cooking oats	500 mL
1 cup	softened margarine or butter	250 mL
1 1/2 cups	granulated sugar	375 mL
2	eggs	2
1 tsp	vanilla	5 mL
1 cup	raisins	250 mL
1 cup	coarsely chopped cranberries, fresh or frozen	250 mL
1 tbsp	grated orange zest	15 mL

1. In a bowl, mix together flour, baking powder, baking soda, salt and oats.

2. In another bowl, beat margarine and sugar until smooth and creamy. Beat in eggs, one at a time, until well incorporated. Mix in vanilla. Add flour mixture and mix well. Fold in raisins, cranberries and orange zest.

3. Drop by rounded teaspoonfuls (5 mL), about 2 inches (5 cm) apart, onto prepared cookie sheet. Bake in preheated oven for 10 to 12 minutes or until edges are lightly browned. Immediately transfer to wire racks to cool.

**FOOD CHOICE VALUES
PER SERVING
(1 COOKIE)**

1/2 ■ Starch Choice

1/2 ✳ Sugars Choice

1/2 ▲ Fats & Oils
Choice

NUTRIENT ANALYSIS PER SERVING			
Calories	86	Fat, total	4 g
Carbohydrates	13 g	Fat, saturated	1 g
Fiber	1 g	Sodium	69 mg
Protein	1 g	Cholesterol	7 mg

Preheat oven to
350°F (180°C)

Cookie sheet lined
with foil, bright side up

Oatmeal Lace Pennies

1 cup	old-fashioned rolled oats	250 mL
1 cup	granulated sugar	250 mL
3 tbsp	all-purpose flour	45 mL
¼ tsp	baking powder	1 mL
½ tsp	salt	2 mL
1	egg, beaten	1
½ cup	margarine or butter, melted	125 mL
½ tsp	vanilla	2 mL

1. In a bowl, mix together oats, sugar, flour, baking powder and salt.

2. In another bowl, beat egg, margarine and vanilla. Add flour mixture and mix well. (If dough seems too soft, chill for 15 to 20 minutes to firm.)

3. Drop by rounded teaspoonfuls (5 mL), about 2 inches (5 cm) apart, onto prepared cookie sheet. Bake in preheated oven for 8 to 10 minutes. Cool for 2 minutes on foil, then transfer to wire racks to cool completely.

**FOOD CHOICE VALUES
PER SERVING
(1 COOKIE)**

½ ✴ Sugars Choice

½ ▲ Fats & Oils
Choice

NUTRIENT ANALYSIS PER SERVING

Calories	32	Fat, total	2 g
Carbohydrates	4 g	Fat, saturated	1 g
Fiber	0 g	Sodium	32 mg
Protein	0 g	Cholesterol	7 mg

Diced Rhubarb Cookies

Tip
If you are lactose
intolerant, use
lactose-reduced milk
in baking. It can be
substituted for regular
milk and will not
affect the results.

2 cups	all-purpose flour or whole wheat flour or a combination of both	500 mL
2 tsp	baking powder	10 mL
Pinch	salt	Pinch
1 tsp	cinnamon	5 mL
½ tsp	nutmeg	2 mL
½ tsp	cloves	2 mL
½ cup	softened margarine or butter	125 mL
1 cup	lightly packed brown sugar	250 mL
1	egg	1
¼ cup	milk	50 mL
1 cup	diced rhubarb	250 mL
1 cup	chopped walnuts	250 mL

1. In a bowl, combine flour, baking powder, salt, cinnamon, nutmeg and cloves.

2. In another bowl, beat margarine and sugar until smooth and creamy. Beat in egg until well incorporated. Mix in milk. Add flour mixture and beat until smooth. Fold in rhubarb and walnuts until well combined.

3. Drop by rounded teaspoonfuls (5 mL), 2 inches (5 cm) apart, onto prepared cookie sheet. Bake in preheated oven for 18 to 20 minutes or until crisp and lightly browned. Immediately transfer to wire racks to cool.

**FOOD CHOICE VALUES
PER SERVING
(1 COOKIE)**

½ ▣ Starch Choice

½ ✳ Sugars Choice

1 ▲ Fats & Oils
Choice

NUTRIENT ANALYSIS PER SERVING			
Calories	83	Fat, total	4 g
Carbohydrates	11 g	Fat, saturated	2 g
Fiber	0 g	Sodium	48 mg
Protein	1 g	Cholesterol	11 mg

Preheat oven to
350°F (180°C)

Lightly greased
cookie sheet

Whole Wheat Spice Cookies

¼ cup	vegetable oil	50 mL
¼ cup	molasses	50 mL
½ cup	granulated sugar	125 mL
¼ cup	packed brown sugar	50 mL
2	eggs	2
½ cup	whole wheat flour	125 mL
1½ cups	all-purpose flour	375 mL
2 tsp	baking soda	10 mL
¼ tsp	salt	1 mL
1 tsp	ginger	5 mL
1 tsp	cinnamon	5 mL
1 tsp	cloves	5 mL

1. In a bowl, whisk oil, molasses, sugars and eggs until blended.

2. In a large bowl, mix together flours, baking soda, salt, ginger, cinnamon and cloves. Make a well in the center and add the molasses mixture, mixing until thoroughly blended.

3. Drop by teaspoonfuls (5 mL), about 2 inches (5 cm) apart, onto prepared cookie sheets. Bake in preheated oven for 8 to 10 minutes or until cookies are firm to the touch. Cool on sheets for 5 minutes, then transfer to wire racks to cool completely.

**FOOD CHOICE VALUES
PER SERVING
(1 COOKIE)**

½ ■ Starch Choice

½ ✳ Sugars Choice

½ ▲ Fats & Oils Choice

NUTRIENT ANALYSIS PER SERVING			
Calories	65	Fat, total	2 g
Carbohydrates	11 g	Fat, saturated	0 g
Fiber	0 g	Sodium	87 mg
Protein	1 g	Cholesterol	12 mg

Sesame Seed Cookies

Preheat oven to
350°F (180°C)

Lightly greased
cookie sheet

1 1/2 cups	whole wheat flour	375 mL
1 tsp	baking powder	5 mL
1/4 tsp	salt	1 mL
1/4 cup	softened margarine or butter	50 mL
1/4 cup	liquid honey	50 mL
1/4 cup	sesame paste (tahini)	50 mL
1/2 tsp	almond extract	2 mL
1/2 cup	sesame seeds, toasted	125 mL

1. In a bowl, mix together flour, baking powder and salt.

2. In another bowl, beat margarine, honey, sesame paste and almond extract until smooth. Add flour mixture and mix well. Stir in sesame seeds.

3. Shape dough into 1-inch (2.5-cm) balls and place about 2 inches (5 cm) apart on prepared cookie sheet. Using the tines of a fork dipped in flour, flatten, or using your hands, mold into crescent shapes. (Wet your hands first, if using to mold the dough.) Bake in preheated oven for 10 to 12 minutes or until lightly browned. Immediately transfer to wire racks to cool.

**FOOD CHOICE VALUES
PER SERVING
(1 COOKIE)**

1/2 ■ Starch Choice

1 ▲ Fats & Oils Choice

NUTRIENT ANALYSIS PER SERVING			
Calories	87	Fat, total	5 g
Carbohydrates	10 g	Fat, saturated	1 g
Fiber	2 g	Sodium	61 mg
Protein	2 g	Cholesterol	0 mg

Preheat oven to
350°F (180°C)

Cookie sheet, lined with
parchment paper or lightly
greased aluminum foil

Variation

Try with half black
sesame seeds or
flaxseeds and half
white sesame seeds.

Sesame Snap Wafers

⅔ cup	all-purpose flour	150 mL
¼ tsp	baking powder	1 mL
½ cup	margarine or butter, softened	125 mL
1 cup	packed brown sugar	250 mL
1	egg	1
1 tsp	vanilla	5 mL
1¼ cups	sesame seeds, toasted	300 mL

1. Combine flour and baking powder.

2. Cream margarine, sugar, egg and vanilla. Add flour mixture. Mix until combined. Stir in seeds.

3. Drop by teaspoonfuls (5 mL) about 2 inches (5 cm) apart onto prepared cookie sheet. Bake for 6 to 9 minutes or until lightly browned. Cool for 5 minutes on sheet, then transfer to rack and cool completely.

FOOD CHOICE VALUES PER SERVING (1 COOKIE)

1 ✳ Sugars Choice

1 ▲ Fats & Oils Choice

NUTRIENT ANALYSIS PER SERVING			
Calories	43	Fat, total	3 g
Carbohydrates	5 g	Fat, saturated	0 g
Fiber	1 g	Sodium	20 mg
Protein	1 g	Cholesterol	3 mg

Preheat oven to
300°F (150°C)

Cookie sheet, ungreased

Cookie cutters

Tip

Shortbreads are one of
the few cookies that are
altered significantly
when made with
margarine. Although
butter and margarine
contribute the same
amount of total fat to the
recipe, butter contains
more saturated fat than
most soft margarine.

Oatmeal Shortbread

¾ cup	all-purpose flour	175 mL
⅔ cup	oats	150 mL
½ cup	cornstarch	125 mL
½ cup	confectioner's (icing) sugar, sifted	125 mL
¾ cup	butter, softened	175 mL

1. Combine flour, oats, cornstarch and confectioner's sugar in large bowl. With large spoon, blend in butter. Work with hands until soft, smooth dough forms. Shape into ball. If necessary, refrigerate for 30 minutes or until easy to handle.

2. Roll out dough to ¼-inch (5 mm) thickness. Cut into shapes with cookie cutters. Place on cookie sheet. Decorate if desired. Bake for 15 to 25 minutes or until edges are lightly browned. (Time will depend on cookie size.) Cool for 5 minutes on sheet, then transfer to rack and cool completely. Store in tightly covered container.

**FOOD CHOICE VALUES
PER SERVING
(1 COOKIE)**

½ ■ Starch Choice

1 ▲ Fats & Oils
Choice

NUTRIENT ANALYSIS PER SERVING			
Calories	76	Fat, total	5 g
Carbohydrates	8 g	Fat, saturated	3 g
Fiber	0 g	Sodium	45 mg
Protein	1 g	Cholesterol	12 mg

Preheat oven to
325°F (160°C)

Greased cookie sheet

Lemon Almond Biscotti

1¾ cups	all-purpose flour	425 mL
¾ cup	granulated sugar	175 mL
1 tbsp	baking powder	15 mL
2 tbsp	finely grated lemon zest	25 mL
¾ cup	coarsely chopped almonds	175 mL
2	eggs	2
⅓ cup	olive oil	75 mL
1 tsp	vanilla	5 mL
½ tsp	almond extract	2 mL

1. In a bowl, mix together flour, sugar, baking powder, lemon zest and almonds. Make a well in the center.

2. In another bowl, whisk eggs, oil, vanilla and almond extract. Pour into well and mix until a soft, sticky dough forms.

3. Divide dough in half. Shape into two rolls about 10 inches (25 cm) long. Place about 2 inches (5 cm) apart on prepared cookie sheet. Bake in preheated oven for 20 minutes.

4. Cool on sheet for 5 minutes, then cut into slices ½ inch (1 cm) thick. Return to sheet and bake for 10 minutes. Turn slices over and bake for 10 minutes more. Immediately transfer to wire racks.

**FOOD CHOICE VALUES
PER SERVING
(1 COOKIE)**

½ ■ Starch Choice

½ ▲ Fats & Oils Choice

NUTRIENT ANALYSIS PER SERVING			
Calories	78	Fat, total	4 g
Carbohydrates	10 g	Fat, saturated	1 g
Fiber	1 g	Sodium	24 mg
Protein	2 g	Cholesterol	12 mg

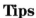
Strawberry-Rhubarb Cobbler

4 cups	chopped fresh rhubarb	1 L
2 cups	sliced strawberries	500 mL
¾ cup	granulated sugar	175 mL
2 tbsp	cornstarch	25 mL
1 tsp	grated orange zest	5 mL

BISCUIT TOPPING

1 cup	all-purpose flour	250 mL
¼ cup	granulated sugar	50 mL
1 ½ tsp	baking powder	7 mL
¼ tsp	salt	1 mL
¼ cup	cold margarine or butter, cut into pieces	50 mL
½ cup	milk	125 mL
1 tsp	vanilla	5 mL
	Additional granulated sugar	

1. Place rhubarb and strawberries in baking dish. In a small bowl, combine sugar, cornstarch and orange zest; sprinkle over fruit and gently toss.

2. Bake in preheated oven for 20 to 25 minutes (increase to 30 minutes if using frozen fruit) until hot and bubbles appear around edges.

3. *Biscuit Topping:* In a bowl, combine flour, sugar, baking powder and salt. Cut in margarine using a pastry blender or fork to make coarse crumbs. In a glass measure, combine milk and vanilla; stir into dry ingredients to make a soft sticky dough.

4. Using a large spoon, drop eight separate spoonfuls of dough onto hot fruit; sprinkle with 2 tsp (10 mL) sugar.

5. Bake in preheated oven for 25 to 30 minutes or until top is golden and fruit is bubbly.

NUTRIENT ANALYSIS PER SERVING			
Calories	246	Fat, total	6 g
Carbohydrates	46 g	Fat, saturated	1 g
Fiber	2 g	Sodium	198 mg
Protein	3 g	Cholesterol	0 mg

Blueberry Flan

1 1/2 cups	all-purpose flour	375 mL
1/4 cup	granulated sugar	50 mL
1 1/2 tsp	baking powder	7 mL
1/4 cup	soft margarine	50 mL
2	egg whites	2
1/4 tsp	almond extract	1 mL
FILLING		
3 cups	fresh blueberries	750 mL
1/3 cup	granulated sugar	75 mL
1 tbsp	all-purpose flour	15 mL
1 tbsp	lemon juice	15 mL
2 tsp	ground cinnamon	10 mL

Tips

Try this recipe using wild or low-bush blueberries when they are in season. They have a delicious and more intense flavor than the cultivated variety.

Blueberries are gaining in popularity because of their antioxidant properties. This delicious flan contains a minimal amount of fat.

1. In a bowl, combine flour, sugar and baking powder; stir in margarine, egg whites and almond extract to form dough. Press into 9-inch (23 cm) flan pan with removable bottom. Freeze for 15 minutes.

2. *Filling:* In a bowl, mix together blueberries, sugar, flour, lemon juice and cinnamon; pour over crust. Bake in preheated oven for 15 minutes. Reduce temperature to 350°F (180°C); bake for 20 to 25 minutes longer. Cool on rack. Refrigerate for at least 1 hour before serving.

This recipe courtesy of Pamela Good and Carrie Roach, Dietitians.

FOOD CHOICE VALUES PER SERVING

1 1/2 ■ Starch Choices

1/2 ◢ Fruit & Vegetable Choice

1 ✳ Sugars Choice

1 ▲ Fats & Oils Choice

NUTRIENT ANALYSIS PER SERVING

Calories	234	Fat, total	6 g
Carbohydrates	42 g	Fat, saturated	1 g
Fiber	2 g	Sodium	135 mg
Protein	4 g	Cholesterol	0 mg

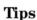

Tips

Most baked custards
have 2 or more eggs.
This custard uses
2% evaporated milk
and 1 egg to create a
slightly softer version.

This is a superb way to
use up all the pumpkin
you scooped out when
making the jack-o'-
lantern for Halloween.
The custard is rich in
vitamin A and calcium
and makes a good finish
for a lighter meal.

Pumpkin Custard

1 cup	2% evaporated milk	250 mL
1 cup	pumpkin purée (not pie filling, if using canned)	250 mL
2 tbsp	granulated sugar	25 mL
1	egg	1
1/4 tsp	ground nutmeg	1 mL
1/4 tsp	ground ginger	1 mL

1. In a blender or food processor, combine milk, pumpkin, sugar, egg and spices. Process until well blended; pour into 4 large or 6 small custard cups. Bake in preheated oven for about 30 minutes or until knife inserted in center comes out clean. Serve warm or cold.

This recipe courtesy of Cynthia Chace, Dietitian.

**FOOD CHOICE VALUES
PER SERVING**

1/2 ◆ 2% Milk Choice

1 ▰ Fruit & Vegetable
Choice

NUTRIENT ANALYSIS PER SERVING			
Calories	82	Fat, total	2 g
Carbohydrates	12 g	Fat, saturated	1 g
Fiber	1 g	Sodium	56 mg
Protein	5 g	Cholesterol	39 mg

Fried Pineapple

Tip
Here's a great recipe for
when you need a
decadent dessert but
don't have time to fuss.
Small amounts of
unsalted butter and
bittersweet chocolate
add 6 g of saturated fat,
so save this for
special occasions.

1	ripe pineapple	1
2 tbsp	sugar	25 mL
2 tbsp	unsalted butter	25 mL
2 tbsp	sultana raisins	25 mL
1 oz	bittersweet chocolate, shaved	25 g
4	sprigs fresh mint	4

1. With a sharp knife cut off top half of pineapple, reserving it for another use. Remove rind from the bottom (sweeter) half and slice pineapple into 4 rounds, each $\frac{1}{2}$ inch (1 cm) thick. Spread sugar on a plate and dredge the pineapple slices in the sugar.

2. In a large frying pan melt butter over high heat until foaming. Add the dredged pineapple slices and fry for 2 minutes. Flip the slices and spread raisins around them; fry for another 2 to 3 minutes until pineapple has browned and raisins are swollen. Remove from heat and transfer one pineapple slice to each of 4 dessert plates, flipping them so the more attractively browned side faces upward. Spoon some raisins onto each plate and top with a bit of the sauce from the pan. Garnish with chocolate shavings and mint. Serve immediately.

FOOD CHOICE VALUES PER SERVING

2½ ◖ Fruit & Vegetable Choices

½ ✳ Sugars Choice

2 ▲ Fats & Oils Choices

NUTRIENT ANALYSIS PER SERVING			
Calories	212	Fat, total	10 g
Carbohydrates	34 g	Fat, saturated	6 g
Fiber	3 g	Sodium	4 mg
Protein	2 g	Cholesterol	16 mg

Strawberry Sorbet

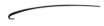
Tips
The perfect low-fat ending to any meal, this sorbet can be made with virtually any fruit. Try raspberries, peaches, blueberries, kiwi fruit, cantaloupe or any other seasonal fruit.

Beating the sorbet during the freezing process helps to keep it from becoming too solid and helps to reduce the formation of ice crystals.

Sorbet is a cool and elegant way to serve fruit and end any meal, particularly during the summer. The strawberries in this recipe are a good source of vitamin C.

1 ½ cups	fresh or frozen unsweetened strawberries	375 mL
2 cups	unsweetened apple juice	500 mL
¼ cup	granulated sugar	50 mL
¼ tsp	ground cinnamon	1 mL
2 tbsp	cold water	25 mL
4 tsp	cornstarch	20 mL

1. Wash and hull fresh strawberries or thaw frozen strawberries. In a blender or food processor, blend strawberries and apple juice until almost smooth.

2. In a medium saucepan over medium heat, cook strawberry mixture, sugar and cinnamon, stirring frequently, for about 5 minutes or until sugar is dissolved. Combine water and cornstarch; stir into hot mixture. Cook for about 3 minutes or until thickened and clear. Chill for 1 hour. Pour into 8-inch (2 L) square pan; cover and freeze for about 3 hours or until firm.

3. Break frozen mixture into chunks; beat with electric mixer at medium speed until fluffy. Transfer to an airtight container and freeze until firm. Transfer from freezer to refrigerator about 15 minutes before serving.

This recipe courtesy of Vicki McKay, Dietitian.

FOOD CHOICE VALUES PER SERVING

1   ◪ Fruit & Vegetable Choice

1   ✱ Sugars Choice

NUTRIENT ANALYSIS PER SERVING

Calories	91	Fat, total	0 g
Carbohydrates	23 g	Fat, saturated	0 g
Fiber	1 g	Sodium	3 mg
Protein	0 g	Cholesterol	0 mg

Lemon Sherbet

½ cup	granulated sugar	125 mL
⅓ cup	lemon juice	75 mL
2 tsp	grated lemon zest	10 mL
2	eggs, separated	2
⅔ cup	skim-milk powder	150 mL
⅔ cup	cold water	150 mL

1. Whisk together sugar, lemon juice, zest and egg yolks; set aside.

2. With an electric mixer, beat egg whites, skim-milk powder and water on high speed for 3 to 5 minutes or until stiff peaks form. Fold in lemon mixture. Pour into 8 small custard cups; cover and freeze for about 3 hours or until firm. Transfer from freezer to refrigerator about 15 minutes before serving.

This recipe courtesy of Joan Gallant, Dietitian.

NUTRIENT ANALYSIS PER SERVING			
Calories	90	Fat, total	1 g
Carbohydrates	17 g	Fat, saturated	0 g
Fiber	0 g	Sodium	47 mg
Protein	4 g	Cholesterol	55 mg

Contributing Authors

The New Vegetarian Gourmet
Byron Ayanoglu
Recipes from this book can be found on pages 20, 22, 23, 36, 111, 117, 120

Simply Mediterranean Cooking
Byron Ayanoglu
A recipe from this book can be found on page 100

The Comfort Food Cookbook
Johanna Burkhard
Recipes from this book can be found on pages 21, 80, 84, 90, 92, 94, 103, 104, 113, 118, 121, 122

Another 250 Best Muffin Recipes
Esther Brody
Recipes from this book can be found on pages 161–165

125 Best Quick Bread Recipes
Donna Washburn and Heather Butt
Recipes from this book can be found on pages 148–160, 166

125 Best Casseroles and One-Pot Meals
Rose Murray
Recipes from this book can be found on pages 51, 65, 73, 81, 82, 93, 98, 105, 124

The 250 Best Cookie Recipes
Esther Brody
Recipes from this book can be found on pages 168, 170–173, 176

300 Best Comfort Food Recipes
Johanna Burkhard
Recipes from this book can be found on pages 30, 31, 35, 41, 42, 58, 96, 108, 112, 119, 126, 127, 140, 177

Dietitians of Canada Cook Great Food
Dietitians of Canada
Recipes from this book can be found on pages 178, 179, 181, 182

Delicious and Dependable
Slow Cooker Recipes
Judith Finlayson
A recipe from this book can be found on page 128

The 150 Best Slow Cooker Recipes
Judith Finlayson
Recipes from this book can be found on pages 38, 89, 99, 114, 115, 129, 131

Fast and Easy Cooking
Johanna Burkhard
Recipes from this book can be found on pages 52, 97

Robert Rose's Favorite Cooking for Kids
Recipes from this book can be found on pages 138, 141, 143, 144

The Robert Rose Book of Classic Pasta
Recipes from this book can be found on pages 49, 54, 60

National Library of Canada Cataloguing in Publication Data

Canada's everyday diabetes choice recipes / edited by Katherine E. Younker.

Published in cooperation with the Canadian Diabetes Association.
Includes index.
ISBN 0-7788-0068-7

1. Diabetes — Diet therapy — Recipes.
I. Younker, Katherine E. II. Canadian Diabetes Association

RC662.C35 2003   641.5'6314   C2002-905888-0

Index

L

Lactose intolerance, 171
Lasagna, roasted vegetable,
    56–57
Leek(s)
  and halibut ragout, 103
  -mango sauce, 53
  pesto over linguine, 47
  white sauce, 54–55
Lemon
  biscotti, 176
  -ginger sauce, 104
  -glazed baby carrots, 121
  sherbet, 182
  yogurt biscuits, 160
Lentils, beef soup with, 33
Linguine
  leek pesto over, 47
  with salmon, leeks and dill, 54–55
Loaf, chicken, 77
Low-fat
  applesauce raisin bread, 152
  herbed beer bread, 148

M

Macaroni
  and cheese
    with beef, 137
    tomato, 51
  chili, turkey, 142
Mango-leek sauce over halibut,
    53
Meat loaf, 80
Meatballs
  pasta casserole, 46–47
  and pasta stew, 134–35
Melizzano despina, 20–21
Mexican hot sauce, 23
Microwave, cooking fish in, 104
Milk, 12
Minerals, 8, 9
Minestrone
  barley, 32
  vegetable, 30
Moors and Christians, 114–15
Muffins
  banana peanut butter, 145
  blueberry wheat germ, 163
  honey whole wheat, 162
  kiwi raspberry, 165
  peanut butter surprise, 164
  tip, 161
  whole wheat, 161

Mushroom(s)
  barley
    pilaf, 127
    soup, 34–35
  risotto, 126–27
  veal paprikash, 92

N

Navy beans, minestrone, 30
New Orleans braised onions, 128
Nutrition, principles, 7–11
Nuts, to toast, 25

O

Oatmeal
  cranberry orange cookies, 169
  lace pennies, 170
  shortbread, 175
  tips, 80
Oats
  blueberry banana bread, 154
  poppy seed bread, 153
  raisin cookies, 168
Oils, 7, 11, 13–14
Onions
  braised, 128
  caramelized, pasta pizza with
    goat cheese and, 59
  with hot sauce, 129
Orange
  broccoli with red pepper, 118
  cranberry oatmeal cookies, 169
  pumpkin snacking cake, 166
  rhubarb bread, 155

P

Paella, 65
Pancakes, Russian blini, 157
Parmesan
  chicken fingers, 140
  sauce, 130–31
Parsnip, carrots and rutabaga,
    lemon-glazed, 121
Pasta
  and bean salad with creamy basil
    dressing, 116–17
  beef and sausage, 48
casserole with meatballs and tomato
    cheese sauce, 46–47
  curried chicken with dried fruit,
    44
Pasta pizza, with goat cheese and
    onions, 59